A

wledge,

essionals

ou are accep

rned to the

Differential Diagnosis in Primary Care

il the date

b

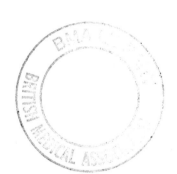

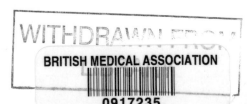

Differential Diagnosis in Primary Care

Nairah Rasul BSc (Hons) MBBS
GP Registrar

Mehmood Syed MBBS DRCOG MRCGP
General Practitioner

WILEY-BLACKWELL
A John Wiley & Sons, Ltd., Publication

BMJ|Books

Library of Congress Cataloging-in-Publication Data

Rasul, Nairah.
   Differential diagnosis in primary care / by Nairah Rasul, Mehmood Syed.
     p. ; cm.
   Includes index.
   ISBN 978-1-4051-8036-8 1. Diagnosis, Differential. 2. Primary care (Medicine) I. Syed, Mehmood. II. Title.
   [DNLM: 1. Diagnosis, Differential. 2. Primary Health Care--methods. 3. Signs and Symptoms. WB 141.5 R213d 2009]
   RC71.5.R375 2009
   616.07'5--dc22

A catalogue record for this book is available from the British Library.

Set in 10/13 pt Frutiger by Newgen Imaging Systems (P) Ltd, Chennai, India
Printed in Singapore by Ho Printing Singapore Pte Ltd

1 2009

Contents

Acknowledgements

We would like to thank Dr Knut Schroeder for his careful review of each of our chapters and Dr Conor O'Doherty for supplying the dermatology pictures used in the book.

Preface

The ability of a doctor to differentiate between diseases on the basis of symptoms and signs alone is fundamental to any good medical consultation. All too often, however, doctors rely heavily on expensive and unnecessary investigations where good history-taking and careful examination would suffice. The typical primary care physician rarely has access to rapid test results and is often forced to rely on clinical judgement alone. Navigating the potential minefield of missed diagnoses and inappropriate referrals can be extremely daunting for both uninitiated trainees and experienced practitioners alike.

The central purpose of this book is to act as a guide to the common symptoms encountered in everyday primary care consultations. By focusing on the key features in the history and examination which differentiate diseases, we hope the text will serve to narrow the list of possible diagnoses from a vast number to a manageable few.

For ease of reference, the majority of the book has been divided into anatomical chapters. Additional systems-based chapters and a 'Miscellaneous' chapter have been included for symptoms which do not fit neatly into an anatomical classification. Each chapter is divided into symptoms seen commonly in primary care. Under each of these symptom-headings, the most likely diagnoses are listed in descending order of likelihood, together with their differentiating features. Prevalence data have been used, where available, to order the diagnoses. However, where such data were unavailable, the authors have relied on their own judgement and experience. Significant conditions, together with key facts, are listed in red text to highlight their importance.

For any symptom encountered in the primary care consultation, consideration must be given to physical, social and psychological factors. This book has focused on the established physical and psychological causes of symptoms, but cannot address the unique social factors which influence a presentation. The clinician faced with these problems must remember to consider these social aspects, once the potential physical and psychological factors have been sufficiently excluded.

In preparing this book, we have deliberately avoided any discussion of management, as rapid developments in healthcare will make any such text virtually obsolete within months of publication. The availability of internet access also means that up-to-date guidance on management is readily accessible and is therefore unnecessary in this text.

We hope the book will help to clarify the key variables in decision-making for all those embarking on a primary care rotation regardless of their level of training. We also hope the book will be evidently useful to the more experienced physician, as an indispensable aide-mémoire.

Dr Mehmood Syed
Dr Nairah Rasul

List of Abbreviations and Symbols

Red text	**Indicates emergency conditions**	CAD	Coronary artery disease
≈	Approximately	CBD	Common bile duct obstruction
>	Greater than	CCF	Congestive cardiac failure
<	Less than	CD4	Cluster of differentiation 4
≥	Greater than or equal to	CF	Cystic fibrosis
≤	Less than or equal to	CFTR	Cystic fibrosis transmembrane conductance regulator
±	Present or absent	CHD	Coronary heart disease
−ve: +ve	negative and positive, respectively	CIN	Cervical intraepithelial neoplasia
		CIS	Carcinoma in situ
A2	Aortic component of second heart sound	CJD	Creutzfeldt-Jakob disease
		CLL	Chronic lymphocytic anaemia
AAA	Abdominal aortic aneurysm	CMV	Cytomegalovirus
AB	Antibody	CN	Cranial nerve
ACE	Angiotensin-converting enzyme	CNS	Central nervous system
ACS	Acute coronary syndrome	COCP	Combined oral contraceptive pill
ACTH	Adrenocorticotrophic hormone	COPD	Chronic obstructive pulmonary disease
ADH	Antidiuretic hormone	CRF	Chronic renal failure
ADL	Activities of daily living	CSF	Cerebrospinal fluid
AF	Atrial fibrillation	CT	Computer tomography
AIDS	Acquired immunodeficiency syndrome	CVA	Cerebrovascular accident
AMA	Anti-mitochondrial antibody		
AML	Acute myeloid leukaemia	DIC	Disseminated intravascular coagulation
ANA	Antinuclear antibody	DIP	Distal interphalangeal
AR	Aortic regurgitation	DKA	Diabetic ketoacidosis
ARF	Acute renal failure	DM	Diabetes mellitus
AS	Aortic stenosis	dsDNA	Double-stranded deoxyribonucleic acid
AV	Atrioventricular	DVLA	Driving and vehicle licensing agency
		DVT	Deep vein thrombosis
BCC	Basal cell carcinoma		
BCG	Bacillus Calmette-Guérin	*E. coli*	*Escherichia coli*
BMI	Body mass index	ECG	Electrocardiogram
BP	Blood pressure	eGFR	Estimated glomerular filtration rate
BPH	Benign prostatic hypertrophy	ENT	Ear, nose and throat
bpm	Beats per minute	ERP	Endoscopic retrograde cholangiopancreatography
BSE	Bovine spongiform encephalopathy	ET	Eustachian tube
BXO	Balanitis xerotica obliterans		
		F	Female
C. coli	*Campylobacter coli*	FEV	Forced expiratory volume
C. jejuni	*Campylobacter jejuni*		

FH	Family history		LIF	Left iliac fossa
fl	Femtolitre		LMN	Lower motor neurone
FSH	Follicle-stimulating hormone		LN	Lymph node
FVC	Forced vital capacity		LRTI	Lower respiratory tract infection
			LV	Left ventricular
GBM	Glomerular basement membrane		LVF	Left ventricular failure
GCS	Glasgow coma scale		LVH	Left ventricular hypertrophy
GI	Gastrointestinal		LoC	Loss of consciousness
GN	Glomerulonephritis		LUQ	Left upper quadrant
GORD	Gastro-oesophageal reflux disease			
GTN	Glyceryl trinitrate		M	Male
GU	Genitourinary		MCP	Metacarpophalangeal
GUM	Genitourinary medicine		MCV	Mean cell volume
G6PD	Glucose-6 phosphate deficiency		MEN	Multiple endocrine neoplasia
			M:F	Male to female ratio
h	Hours		MI	Myocardial infarction
H. pylori	*Helicobacter pylori*		Mins	Minutes in this list
HBsAg	Hepatitis B Surface antigen		MR	Mitral regurgitation
HBV	Hepatitis B virus		MS	Multiple sclerosis
HCC	Hepatocellular carcinoma		MTP	Metatarsal–phalangeal joint
hCG	Human chorionic gonadotrophin			
HCV	Hepatitis C virus		NaCl	Sodium chloride
HDL	High-density lipoprotein		NAI	Non-accidental injury
HIV	Human immunodeficiency virus		NSAID	Non-steroidal anti-inflammatory drug
HOCM	Hypertrophic obstructive cardiomyopathy		OA	Osteoarthritis
HONK	Hyperosmolar non-ketotic coma		P2	Pulmonary component of second heart sound
HPV	Human papilloma virus		PBC	Primary biliary cirrhosis
HRT	Hormone replacement therapy		PCOS	Polycystic ovarian syndrome
HSV	Herpes simplex virus		PCP	Pneumocystis carinii pneumonia
HR	Heart rate		PCT	Porphyria cutanea tarda
5-HT	5-hydroxytryptamine		PE	Pulmonary embolism
			PEFR	Peak expiratory flow rate
IBD	Inflammatory bowel disease		PHT	Pulmonary hypertension
IBS	Irritable bowel syndrome		PID	Pelvic inflammatory disease
ICP	Intracranial pressure		PIP	Proximal interphalangeal
IDDM	Insulin-independent diabetes mellitus		PKD	Polycystic kidney disease
Ig	Immunoglobulin		PMT	Premenstrual tension
IHD	Ischaemic heart disease		PND	Paroxysmal nocturnal dyspnoea
i.m.	Intramuscular		POP	Progesterone-only pill
IP	Interphalangeal		PR	Per rectum
IUCD	Intrauterine contraceptive device		PSA	Prostate-specific antigen
IUGR	Intrauterine growth restriction		PSC	Primary sclerosing cholangitis
i.v.	Intravenous		PV	Per vaginam
IVDU	Intravenous drug user		PVD	Peripheral vascular disease
JVP	Jugular venous pressure		QoL	Quality of life
KS	Kaposi's sarcoma		RA	Rheumatoid arthritis
L	Left		RAD	Right axis deviation
LA	Left atrium		RBBB	Right bundle branch block
LH	Luteinizing hormone		RIF	Right iliac fossa

RNA	Ribonucleic acid
ROM	Range of movement
RSV	Respiratory syncytial virus
RTA	Road traffic accident
RUQ	Right upper quadrant
RV	Right ventricle
RVF	Right ventricular failure
RVH	Right ventricular hypertrophy
S1, S2, S3	First, second and third heart sounds
SA	Sino-atrial node
SCC	Squamous cell carcinoma
SE	South East
Secs	Seconds
SHBG	Sex hormone–bonding globulin
SLE	Systemic lupus erythematosus
SOB	Shortness of breath
SOL	Space-occupying lesion
STI	Sexually transmitted infection
SVT	Supraventricular tachycardia

TB	Tuberculosis
TCA	Tricyclic anti-depressants
TIA	Transient ischaemic attack
TM	Tympanic membrane
TMJ	Temporomandibular joint
TSH	Thyroid-stimulating hormone
TURP	Transurethral resection of prostate
UMN	Upper motor neurone
URTI	Upper respiratory tract infection
UTI	Urinary tract infection
UV	Ultraviolet
VF	Ventricular fibrillation
VSD	Ventricular septal defect
VT	Ventricular tachycardia
WCC	White cell count
Wks	Weeks
Yrs	Years

Chapter 1
Head and Neck

Facial pain or swelling

Diagnosis	Background	Key symptoms	Key signs	Additional information
Acute sinusitis (Rhinosinusitis)	Paranasal sinus inflammation Nose frequently involved Acute bacterial infection lasts between 10 and 30 days Common causes: *Haemophilus influenzae* and *Streptococcus* Common risk factors: URTI, smoking, asthma, allergy, DM, swimming, dental infection	*≥2 of the following lasting <12 wks:* Blocked nose Nasal discharge/post-nasal drip Facial pain or pressure Reduction or loss of smell ± Headache ± Malaise ± Upper toothache	Tenderness over sinuses Normal respiratory examination Facial pain worse on stooping ± Fever	
Ophthalmic shingles (See Painful eye)				
Temporal arteritis (Giant cell arteritis)	Age >50 yrs ≥25% also have polymyalgia rheumatica	Unilateral headache Worse at night Jaw claudication Acute visual disturbance in one eye Malaise	Scalp tenderness ± Optic neuritis (swollen optic disc, painful eye movements, visual field defect) ± Retinal artery thrombosis (pale retina, red fovea and arteriolar narrowing)	Requires immediate high-dose steroids Refer to ophthalmology if visual symptoms
Trigeminal neuralgia	Chronic debilitating condition Neuropathic disorder of V nerve Commonly age >50 yrs M<F Causes include: Vascular nerve compression, tumour, idiopathic Intermittent pains last days to months Often recurrent ≈4% cases associated with MS	Paroxysms of severe stabbing pains Last a second up to 2 mins Occurs day and night Commonly affects mandibular and maxillary areas Pain triggered by touch, facial movement, cold	Typically unilateral Pain affects ≥1 trigeminal divisions No facial neurological deficit	Exclude dental pathology
Temporomandibular joint dysfunction	Abnormal jaw function Jaw anatomy may be normal or abnormal Onset early adolescence/ adulthood Can persist into middle-age M:F ratio: ≈1:4 Associated with bruxism and/or joint disease (e.g. arthritis)	Facial pain Headache Painful jaw	Crepitus on jaw movement Restricted jaw movement Painful jaw movement ± Depression or anxiety	
Parotitis	Causes: Bacterial infection, dehydration (e.g. post-op), poor oral hygiene	Unilateral facial pain and swelling	Unilateral swelling at the angle of the jaw Firm tender swelling Erythema ± Fever	Pain or swelling on eating indicates calculi

Differential Diagnosis in Primary Care, 1st edition. By Nairah Rasul and Mehmood Syed. Published 2009 by Blackwell Publishing, ISBN: 978-1-4051-8036-8

Diagnosis	Background	Key symptoms	Key signs	Additional information
Mumps	Often no Mumps immunisation	Prodromal malaise	Fever Unilateral or bilateral parotid swelling Tenderness ± Unilateral orchitis a few days later	Notifiable disease Complications: Meningitis, pancreatitis, myocarditis, arthritis
Angioedema	Allergen factor often present (e.g. food, drugs, insect bite)	Acute onset Pruritis	Bilateral facial swelling Facial erythema Urticaria ± Lip and tongue swelling	Airway compromise warrants adrenaline and emergency admission
Erysipelas	Caused by beta-haemolytic *Streptococcus* skin innoculation Peak age 60–80 yrs Risk factors: Inflammatory dermatoses, skin trauma, nasopharyngeal infection, dermatophyte infections, poor hygiene, DM, alcohol abuse, immunodeficiency, nephrotic syndrome	Prodromal malaise and chills Followed by acute symptoms: Pruritis Skin burning Tender skin Red skin patch Enlarges over 3–6 days Affects face or legs Anorexia Fatigue Arthralgia	High-grade fever >39°C Shiny plaque Deep erythema Sharply demarcated Raised edges Skin oedema Indurated Warm and tender skin ± Vesicles and bullae	Compared with cellulitis, erysipelas is more sharply demarcated and has raised edges
Parotid tumour	≈90% are benign (pleomorphic adenoma)	Unilateral facial lump Slowly enlarges Pain worse on jaw movement	No fever Superficial mobile mass at angle of mandible	Facial palsy suggests malignancy
Superior vena cava obstruction	≈75% due to lung cancer	Shortness of breath Headache worse on stooping	Swelling of face, neck, upper limb Non-pulsatile dilated veins in neck and chest	Requires urgent investigation

Headache

Diagnosis	Background	Key symptoms	Key signs	Additional information
Tension headache	Episodic or chronic (>15 days per month) Associated with emotional stress	Generalised pressure/tightness around head Radiation to or from neck	Normal neurological examination	Exclude musculoskeletal problems (e.g. cervicogenic headache)
Migraine	Late teens to 50s M:F ratio:: ≈1:3		Normal examination between attacks	
Subtypes:				
Classical migraine	Aura present	Unilateral throbbing headache Aura precedes headache *Visual aura*: Homonymous hemianopia Scintillating scotoma "Zigzag" of flashing lights (fortification spectrum)		Aura can be visual, sensory, involve speech or limbs Stop COCP
Common migraine	Aura absent	No aura ≥5 headaches lasting 4–72 h Nausea/vomiting or Photophobia and phonophobia *Plus ≥2 of the following:* Unilateral headache Pulsating nature Affects QoL Aggravated by routine activity		Look for triggers (e.g. diet, stress)

Diagnosis	Background	Key symptoms	Key signs	Additional information
Acute sinusitis (Rhinosinusitis)	Paranasal sinus inflammation Nose frequently involved Acute bacterial infection lasts between 10 and 30 days Common causes: *Haemophilus influenzae* and *Streptococcus* Common risk factors: URTI, smoking, asthma, allergy, DM, swimming, dental infection	≥2 of the following lasting <12 wks: Blocked nose Nasal discharge/post-nasal drip Facial pain or pressure Reduction or loss of smell ± Headache ± Malaise ± Upper toothache	Tenderness over sinuses Normal respiratory examination Facial pain worse on stooping ± Fever	
Post-concussion syndrome	Common causes: RTA, sports injury, fall, assault Full recovery should be achieved within 2 wks	Onset symptoms days after minor head trauma Persistent mild headache Not getting worse Dizziness Memory loss (retrograde or anterograde) Low mood Poor concentration Irritability Nausea with no vomiting	GCS 15/15 No confusion Normal gait and balance No visual problems No focal neurology (e.g. limb weakness)	Discharge from nose or ear suggests CSF leak from basal skull fracture Refer immediately
Medication	Chronic analgesia use: NSAID, paracetamol, codeine, ergotamine Medication side-effects: GTN, nifedipine, substance withdrawal	Onset symptoms after taking medication	Normal neurological examination	
Temporal arteritis (Giant cell arteritis)	Age >50 yrs ≥25% also have polymyalgia rheumatica	Unilateral headache Worse at night Jaw claudication Acute visual disturbance in one eye Malaise	Scalp tenderness ± Optic neuritis (swollen optic disc, painful eye movements, visual field defect) ± Retinal artery thrombosis (pale retina, red fovea and arteriolar narrowing)	Requires immediate high-dose steroids Refer to ophthalmology if visual symptoms
Cluster headache	Age >20 yrs M:F ratio: ≈6:1 Recurrent annual event	Daily symptoms for 6–12 wks Severe unilateral headache Retro-orbital pain Worse at night	Unilateral Red watery eye Ptosis Rhinorrhoea or nasal blockage	
Malignant hypertension	BP >200/130 mmHg Young adults Commonly Afro-Caribbean Other risk factors include: Obesity, smoking, DM	Visual disturbance	Bilateral retinal haemorrhages Encephalopathy *Abnormal urinalysis:* Proteinuria	Admit for BP control
Intracranial tumour	<1% of all headaches Age >50 yrs	New onset headache Worse in the morning Progressively worsening Nausea/vomiting Personality change (e.g. disinhibition) ± Seizures (≤50%)	Drowsiness Falling pulse and rising BP (Cushing's reflex) Papilloedema (≈50%) Focal neurology	Refer for urgent neurology review
Subarachnoid haemorrhage	M<F Causes: Berry aneurysms, arterio-venous malformation, bleeding disorder	Sudden onset occipital headache Severe pain Nausea/vomiting	Neck stiffness Focal neurology Collapse ± LoC *Positive Kernig's sign:* Pain and resistance on passive knee extension with hips flexed	Emergency admission

Diagnosis	Background	Key symptoms	Key signs	Additional information
Meningitis	Common viruses: Echovirus, herpes simplex and zoster, coxsackie, HIV, measles, influenza Common bacteria: *Streptococcus pneumoniae, Neiserria meningitidis, Haemophilus influenzae* type B, *Listeria* Elderly and young age <2 yrs are particularly susceptible	Acute onset of symptoms Frontal headache Nausea/vomiting Severe leg pains Neck pain ± Non-blanching purple skin rash	Fever Cold peripheries Drowsiness Irritability Neck stiffness Photophobia Papilloedema (raised ICP) ± Petechial rash *Positive Kernig's sign:* Pain and resistance on passive knee extension with hips flexed *Positive Brudzinski's sign:* Hips flex on bending head forward	Notifiable disease DO NOT delay antibiotic treatment Petechiae suggest meningococcus or pneumococcus meningitis
Benign intracranial hypertension	Commonly young women Typically obese Often self-limiting	Blurred vision or diplopia	Papilloedema *VI nerve palsy (lateral rectus):* Eye is medially deviated Lateral eye movement not possible Horizontal diplopia on looking out	
Carbon monoxide poisoning	Risk of fits and coma if prolonged exposure	Nausea/vomiting Dizziness Worse when heater or cooking appliance in use Relieved when away from house	Pink skin and oral mucosa Tachypnoea Tachycardia	Check gas appliances and flues
Pre-eclampsia (See Abdominal pain in pregnancy)				

Neck lump

Diagnosis	Background	Key symptoms	Key signs	Additional information
Non-specific reactive lymphadenitis	History of recent URTI infection	URTI symptoms (e.g. sore throat)	Enlarged cervical LN	LN usually reduce 2 wks post-infection
Tonsillitis	Commonly children and young adults	Acute onset Painful swallow Headache	Fever Erythematous tonsils ± white exudate Enlarged and tender anterior cervical LN	Consider ENT referral if ≥5 episodes per year
Glandular fever (Infectious mononucleosis)	Caused by Epstein Barr virus Commonly teenagers and young adults Droplet spread Post-viral fatigue is common	Often few symptoms Sore throat >1 wk Prolonged fatigue or malaise Transient non-itchy rash	Fine macular rash Transient bilateral upper eyelid oedema Palatal petechiae Generalised LN Splenomegaly (10%–30%)	Avoid amoxicillin Avoid contact sports for 6 wks due to risk of splenic rupture
Sebaceous cyst (Epidermoid cyst)	Proliferation of epidermal cells in the dermis Benign Slow growth Commonly young adults M>F Common sites: Face, trunk, neck, extremities, scalp Often resolves spontaneously Often recurs if not excised	Painless lump(s)	Skin-coloured nodule Single or multiple Often round or oval Variable in size Firm subcutaneous nodule Central punctum Fixed to skin Not reducible Not pulsatile ± Uninfected foul cheese-like discharge	A tender and erythematous cyst suggests infection
Thyroglossal cyst	Often presents 15–30 yrs of age	Painless neck lump	Smooth midline swelling Moves up on protrusion of tongue	Refer to ENT surgeon as risk of infection

Diagnosis	Background	Key symptoms	Key signs	Additional information
Goitre			Lump moves up with swallowing	
Subtypes:				
Physiological	Causes: Pregnancy, puberty and/or stress	Neck lump	Smooth enlarged thyroid	
Non-toxic simple	Thyroid enlarges to compensate for mild hypothyroidism M<F Causes: Iodine deficiency (rare in UK), familial inborn error of iodine metabolism	Neck lump	Smooth enlarged thyroid Becomes multinodular if untreated	
Non-toxic multinodular (Colloid)	Most common goitre in the UK Mild hypothyroidism	Pressure symptoms if large (e.g. dysphagia)	Enlarged irregular thyroid	
Toxic diffuse (Graves' disease)	Young adults M<F Hyperthyroid Due to thyroid autoantibodies	Hyperactivity Sweating Weight loss despite good appetite Heat intolerance	Tachycardia Exophthalmos Lid lag Smooth uniform enlargement of thyroid Fine hand tremor Audible bruit over goitre	
Toxic multinodular	Typically middle-age Hyperthyroid	Insidious onset Palpitations Weight loss Shortness of breath Swollen ankles	Irregular thyroid enlargement Atrial fibrillation Heart failure	
Solitary nodule	May be benign or malignant Hyperthyroid	Asymptomatic or Hyperactivity Sweating Weight loss despite good appetite Heat intolerance	Solitary lump in thyroid *Suspect malignancy if:* History of rapid enlargement Hard nodule Palpable cervical LN Hoarse voice	Clinically difficult to differentiate benign from malignant therefore refer for further investigation
De Quervain's thyroiditis (Acute thyroiditis)	Self-limiting viral infection Usually resolves within 2 wks	Acutely painful thyroid Pain radiates to ears Malaise	Fever Diffuse thyroid enlargement Firm and tender thyroid	Frank thyrotoxicosis is common initially, followed occasionally by post-viral hypothyroidism
Hashimoto's disease (Chronic lymphocytic thyroiditis)	Autoimmune destruction of thyroid Peak age 30–50 yrs M:F ratio: ≈1:15 ≈50% become permanently hypothyroid	Slow-growing neck lump Painless	Thyroid enlargement Non-tender Rubbery and mobile on palpation Initially hyperthyroidsim followed by hypothyroidism	
Postpartum thyroiditis	Affects 5%–10% women up to 12 months postpartum ≈25% become permanently hypothyroid	Fatigue Low mood Weight gain Constipation	Painless thyroid enlargement Coarse skin Dry hair	Exclude postpartum depression
Lymphoma				
Subtypes:				
Non-Hodgkin's	Five times more common than Hodgkin's lymphoma Commonly presents >50 yrs of age M<F Disease may originate from extranodal sites (e.g. GI, skin, chest)	Often asymptomatic or Presents like Hodgkin's	Anaemia Painless LN enlargement Hepatosplenomegaly	
Hodgkin's	Young adults and elderly M:F ratio: ≈2:1 Risk factors: History of infectious mononucleosis, HIV, immunosupression, smoking	*A symptoms:* Asymptomatic or pruritis *B symptoms:* Chronic weight loss >10% in 6 months Fever Night sweats	Cachexia Anaemia Painless LN enlargement (neck, axillae, supraclavicular) Hepatosplenomegaly	B symptoms indicate more extensive disease

Diagnosis	Background	Key symptoms	Key signs	Additional information
Branchial cyst	Congenital Often enlarges post-URTI	Usually painless neck lump	Oval cystic swelling Deep to upper 1/3 of sternocleidomastoid muscle	Refer for excision Recurrent infection increases risk of sinus/fistula
Dermoid cyst	Commonly children	Neck lump Common sites: Periorbital, submental, sublingual	Smooth spherical neck lump Hard on palpation Not attached to skin Usually ≈1 cm in diameter Transilluminant	

Neck pain and stiffness

Diagnosis	Background	Key symptoms	Key signs	Additional information
Spasmodic torticollis (Wry neck)	Occasionally associated with poor posture Often self-limiting	Acute onset Neck pain and stiffness	Spasm of trapezius and sternocleidomastoid muscles Restricted passive and active neck movements ± Neck held flexed away from pain	Exclude neck trauma and upper-limb neurology
Cervical spondylosis	Chronic cervical disc degeneration Disc herniation, calcification and osteophytic outgrowths Age >40 yrs	Gradual onset symptoms Intermittent neck pain and stiffness Radiation to occiput, interscapular, upper limb ± Paraesthesia of arm ± Arm weakness	Usually unilateral Tender neck spine Shoulder joint non-tender on palpation Reduced ROM of neck ± Sensory loss and hyporeflexia of upper limb	
Whiplash injury	History of recent flexion/extension injury (e.g. RTA, sport, fall)	Symptoms occur hours/days post-trauma Neck stiffness ± Pain radiates to head, arms and back	Tender or tense trapezius muscle Pain on neck movement Reduced ROM of neck No upper limb neurology	Anxiety, depression and litigation can all delay recovery
Cervical disc prolapse	Due to neck trauma or degenerative disease Symptoms are acute in trauma and gradual in degenerative disease C6 and C7 are most commonly affected Often resolves spontaneously	Neck stiffness Worse on coughing or straining Relieved by lying down Shooting pains radiate to occiput, interscapular or upper limb Paraesthesia in distal limb	Usually unilateral Reduced ROM of neck Neck pain may be absent *Radiculopathy:* Upper-limb wasting Proximal limb weakness Reduced sensation in C6 and C7 dermatomes Reduced or absent biceps and triceps reflex	
Cervical cord compression	Common causes: Neck trauma, malignancy, prolapsed cervical disc LMN signs at level of lesion UMN signs below level of lesion	Paraesthesia in arms and hands Upper limb weakness	Tender cervical vertebrae Reduced grip/power in affected upper limb Reduced sensation in upper limb Lower limb spasticity and sphincter disturbance (late sign)	Emergency neurosurgical referral

Chapter 2
Ophthalmology

Eyelid swelling

Diagnosis	Background	Key symptoms	Key signs	Additional information
Blepharitis	Chronic eyelid inflamation Occasionally associated with infection Risk factors: Seborrhoeic dermatitis, atopic eczema, acne rosacea	Tired and sore eyes Gritty sensation Worse in the morning Crusting of lid margin	Often bilateral Crusting around base of lashes (colarettes) Injection of lid margins Meibomian glands covered with small oil globules	
Hordeolum externum (Stye)	Staphylococcal abscess of lash follicle Commonly children Often self-limiting	Acute onset Painful eyelid lump	Lid swelling points outwards Tender lid margin	
Meibomian cyst (Chalazion)	Chronic sterile lipogranulomatous lesion of the meibomian gland Risk factors: Acne rosacea and seborrhoeic dermatitis Usually resolves within 6 months	Painless swelling within eyelid Gradually enlarges	Upper or lower-lid lump Round firm lesion Points inwards towards conjunctiva Non-tender	Pain suggests an infected chalazion (hordeolum internum)
Periorbital cellulitis (Preseptal cellulitis)	Inflammation and infection of the lid only Orbit not involved Commonly children Risk factors: Recent local trauma (e.g. insect bites, laceration), paranasal sinus infection, URTI More prevalent in winter months	Erythema and swelling of lid and periorbital region Painful	Unilateral Lid tenderness Tense eyelid oedema (eye may remain closed) Erythema Painless eye movements Normal visual acuity ± Mild fever ± Mild injection of sclera	
Orbital cellulitis (See Painful eye)				

Differential Diagnosis in Primary Care, 1st edition. By Nairah Rasul and Mehmood Syed. Published 2009 by Blackwell Publishing, ISBN: 978-1-4051-8036-8

Gradual loss of vision

Diagnosis	Background	Key symptoms	Key signs	Additional information
Diabetic retinopathy	Poorly controlled DM with hypertension			
Stages:				
Grade I Background retinopathy		Largely asymptomatic	Microaneurysms (dots) Haemorrhages (flame and dot) Hard exudates (yellow patches)	
Grade II Maculopathy		Potential loss of central vision	Macula oedema Hard exudates (yellow patches)	
Grade III Pre-proliferative retinopathy		Vision largely unaffected	Cotton wool spots Venous dilatation and loops Large blot haemorrhages	
Grade IV Proliferative retinopathy		High risk of loss in vision	New vessel formation on optic disc and retina	May be complicated by retinal detachment and/or secondary glaucoma Refer for laser therapy
Cataract	Commonly >65 yrs age Risk factors: DM, chronic steroid use, ocular trauma, radiation exposure, advancing age Can be congenital	Painless loss of vision Glare in sunlight Difficulty with near vision (e.g. reading)	Unilateral or bilateral Reduced visual acuity Cataract appears black or white against a red reflex Normal pupillary reflex	In infants, a white reflex or absent red reflex warrants an urgent ophthalmology review to exclude cataract and retinoblastoma
Chronic open angle glaucoma	Prevalence increase >65 yrs age Common and more severe in Afro-Carribeans ± Positive family history	Largely asymptomatic in early stages Progressive loss of peripheral vision later	Usually bilateral Abnormally large cup–disc ratio Visual field defect Arcuate scotoma (late sign)	
Dry age-related macular degeneration	Progressive irreversible disease Affects central vision only Age >50 yrs Risk factors: Caucasian, smoking	Steady decline in central vision Difficulty reading small print Difficulty making out people's faces ± Micro/macropsia	Bilateral (often one eye is more severely affected) Discrete yellow macular (Drusen) deposits Scotoma Normal peripheral field vision	Neovascular membrane can develop, causing sudden onset distortion of straight lines and reduced visual acuity. This warrants emergency referral
Retinal detachment	Commonly 40–70 yrs age Risk factors: High myopia, ocular trauma, post-cataract surgery, DM	Prodromal flashing lights (indicates vitreous detachment) Gradual or sudden visual impairment "Like a curtain over the eye" Painless ± Floaters in the peripheral vision	Pink/greyish retina ballooning forwards ± Reduced visual acuity ± Visual field defect	Reduced visual acuity indicates macula detachment. Successful surgery within 24 h of detachment confers a good prognosis Unlike a TIA, visual loss does not resolve spontanoeusly
Pituitary tumour	Mostly benign	Headache worse on waking Loss of peripheral vision Endocrine symptoms	Bitemporal hemianopia ± Squint (ocular palsy)	Endocrine symptoms vary according to the hormone involved
Retinitis pigmentosa	Gradual deterioration in light-sensitive cells of retina Typical onset 10–30 yrs age Inherited condition X-linked recessive is the most severe form Associated deafness indicates other related syndromes (e.g. Usher, Alport syndrome)	Poor night vision/accomodation Loss of peripheral vision ± Loss of central vision (late sign)	Clumps of black/brown retinal flecks ("bone-spicule") pigmentation) Disc pallor Attenuation of retinal arterioles	

Sudden loss of vision

Diagnosis	Background	Key symptoms	Key signs	Additional information
Migraine (See Headache)				
Vitreous haemorrhage	Retinal vessel haemorrhage into the vitreous humour Common causes: Proliferative diabetic retinopathy, retinal tear, posterior vitreous detachment, ocular trauma	Painless Other symptoms vary according to degree of haemorrhage *Small haemorrhage:* Floaters *Large haemorrhage:* Significant loss of vision	Reduced visual acuity Absent red reflex Loss of fundus detail with red floating debris	Requires urgent ophthalmology referral
Retinal artery occlusion	Commonly elderly Risk factors: IHD, carotid artery stenosis, AF, aortic/mitral valve disease, hypertension	Painless Partial or total visual loss in one eye Visual loss may be transient (*Amaurosis fugax*) or permanent	Unilateral Grossly reduced visual acuity Relative afferent pupillary defect Arteriolar narrowing Pale and oedematous retina ± "Cherry red spot" at fovea (central artery occlusion)	Exclude vasculitic causes (e.g. temporal ateritis)
Retinal vein occlusion	Age >50 yrs Risk factors: Hyperviscosity syndromes, glaucoma, vasculitis, DM, smoking, hypertension	Painless Partial or total visual loss in one eye	Unilateral Reduced visual acuity Relative afferent pupillary defect Extensive "storm-like" retinal haemorrhages Cotton wool spots Engorged veins	Requires urgent ophthalmology referral Complications are common (e.g. retinal neovascularisation and secondary glaucoma)
Primary angle closure glaucoma (See Painful eye)				
Optic neuritis	Young adults M<F Often precipitated by viral infection or immunisation in children Spontaneous recovery often occurs in 3–4 wks ≈50% adult cases develop MS	Acute loss of vision over hours/ days Vision may improve gradually Painful eye movements Reduced colour discrimination (dyschromatopsia)	≈70% adult cases are unilateral Reduced visual acuity Relative afferent pupillary defect Visual field defect (e.g. scotoma) ± Swollen optic disc (papillitis)	Papillitis indicates optic head involvement
Temporal ateritis (See Headache)				
Wet (exudative) age-related macular degeneration	Sub-retinal neovascularisation Age >50 yrs Risk factors: Caucasian, smoking	Sudden profound central vision loss Distortion of straight lines (e.g. door, window frames)	Bilateral One eye more severely affected Sub-retinal haemorrhages Macular scarring in late disease (thick yellow patches)	Emergency referral to exclude a treatable condition

Painful eye

Diagnosis	Background	Key symptoms	Key signs	Additional information
Foreign body	History of foreign body striking eye	Vary depending on degree of trauma Watery eye Blurred vision	Eyelid eversion may identify foreign body	Exclude corneal abrasion with fluorescein staining
Non-infective corneal ulcer	History of corneal trauma Risk factor: Contact lens wear	Severe eye pain Worse on waking Watery eye	Red watery eye Photophobia	Emergency referral
Keratitis	Inflammation of the cornea Bacterial, fungal or viral cause Risk factors for bacterial keratitis: Contact lens wear, dry eyes, trauma, prolonged use of topical steroids	Severe gritty eye pain Blurred vision	Circumcorneal injection Hazy cornea Purulent discharge Photophobia Reduced visual acuity ± White/yellow level of pus in anterior chamber (hypopyon)	Urgent ophthalmology review due to risk of ulceration

Diagnosis	Background	Key symptoms	Key signs	Additional information
Keratoconjunctivitis sicca (Dry eye syndrome)	Common in elderly	Symptoms worse at end of day Gritty burning painful eyes Photophobia	*Primary Sjögren's:* Dry eyes Dry mouth Dry cough Enlarged parotids Or *Secondary Sjögrens:* As above plus Autoimmune disease (e.g. RA, SLE)	Exclude antihistamine and anticholinergic use
Ophthalmic shingles	Reactivation of varicella zoster virus Age >50 yrs and/or immunocompromised	Nausea Malaise Facial pain, tingling or numbness precedes rash	Unilateral Rash in ophthalmic division of trigeminal nerve Tenderness Maculopapular rash becomes vesicular before crusting ± Keratitis ± Iritis ± Glaucoma	Nose tip involvement (Hutchinson's sign) indicates high risk of orbital involvement
Primary angle closure glaucoma (Acute glaucoma)	Age >40 yrs M<F Risk factor: Hypermetropia Attacks may be precipitated by pupil dilatation (e.g. dim light)	Acute onset symptoms Unilateral severe eye pain Watery eye Blurred vision ± Haloes around lights ± Nausea ± Abdominal pain	Circumcorneal injection Hazy cornea Pupil fixed, oval and semi-dilated Reduced visual acuity	Emergency referral
Iritis (Anterior uveitis)	Usually idiopathic Associated with systemic disease: Ankylosing spondylitis, Reiter's disease, IBD, psoriasis, Behcet's disease, sarcoidosis	Acute onset symptoms Unilateral eye pain Watery eye Blurred vision Photophobia	Circumcorneal injection Irregular pupil (posterior synechiae) Reduced visual acuity Consensual photophobia ± Anterior chamber pus (hypopyon)	Emergency referral Only prescribe topical steroids under specialist supervision
Arc eye	Inadequate eye protection against UV exposure Usually resolves within 36 h Common in: Welders, mountaineers, sunbed users, skiers, sailors	History of recent UV exposure Severe eye pains 6–8 h later Foreign body sensation Blepharospasm Watery eyes	Normal eye examination	
Scleritis (See Red eye)				
Periorbital cellulitis (Preseptal cellulitis)	Inflammation and infection of the lid only Orbit not involved Commonly children Risk factors: Recent local trauma (e.g. insect bites, laceration), paranasal sinus infection, URTI More prevalent in winter months	Erythema and swelling of lid and periorbital region Painful	Unilateral Lid tenderness Tense eyelid oedema (eye may remain closed) Erythema Painless eye movements Normal visual acuity ± Mild fever ± Mild injection of sclera	
Orbital cellulitis	Inflammation and infection of the orbit and lid Infection usually spreads from paranasal sinuses, commonly ethmoid More prevalent in winter months	Acute onset eyelid swelling Severe eye pain Blurred vision Malaise	Unilateral Fever Lid erythema and oedema Proptosis Double vision Reduced visual acuity Ophthalmoplegia	Emergency admission

Ptosis

Diagnosis	Background	Key symptoms	Key signs	Additional information
Third nerve palsy (Oculomotor nerve palsy)	Associated with central nervous lesion	Double vision Eyelid almost shut	Partial ptosis Impaired eye movement superiorly, inferiorly and medially Diplopia ± Dilated pupil	Pupil sparing suggests ischaemia or DM Urgent referral to a neurologist
Horner's syndrome	Causes include: Congenital lesion, Pancoast's tumour, multiple sclerosis	Vary depending on underlying cause	Partial ptosis Anhidrosis of forehead Pupillary meiosis Enophthalmos	Requires a neurology referral
Myasthenia Gravis	Acquired condition Antibody-mediated autoimmune disorder ≈15% associated with thymoma ≈75% associated with thymic hyperplasia Precipitating factors include: Pregnancy, infection, drugs	Muscular fatigue Common muscles involved: Extra-ocular muscles, limbs, bulbar and/or respiratory	Asymmetrical diplopia or ptosis Rapid muscle fatigue on exercise Shoulder girdle weakness > pelvic girdle weakness Normal tone, reflexes and sensation ± Facial weakness ± Dysarthria	Respiratory muscle involvement requires emergency airway management
Dystrophia myotonica	Autosomal dominant inheritance Commonest muscular dystrophy Usual onset 15–40 yrs age Slowly progressive	Progressive muscle weakness	Reduced muscle power Myotonia of face and limbs Symmetrical ptosis Normal pupils Absent limb reflexes ± Frontal baldness ± Cataract ± Infertility ± Mental impairment	

Red eye

Diagnosis	Background	Key symptoms	Key signs	Additional information
Conjunctivitis				
Subtypes:				
Bacterial	Pathogens include: *Staphylococcus, Streptococcus, Haemophilus* Highly contagious Often self-limiting within a few days	Unilateral or bilateral sore eyes Sticky eyes on waking Gritty sensation	Injected conjunctiva Purulent discharge Normal visual acuity	Can be complicated by keratitis
Viral	Commonly due to Adenovirus Highly contagious Often self-limiting within 1–2 wks	Unilateral or bilateral sore eyes Sticky eyes on waking Gritty sensation	Injected conjunctiva Watery discharge Pre-auricular LN Lid oedema Normal visual acuity	Can be complicated by keratitis
Allergic	History of atopy Seasonal variation Can be precipitated by allergen exposure	Watery and itchy eyes	Bilateral Conjunctival injection and swelling "Cobblestone" appearance under upper lid in chronic allergy ± Photophobia	
Chlamydial inclusion conjunctivitis	Caused by *Chlamydia trachomatis* (serotypes D to K) Commonly young adults or neonates Incubation up to 1 wk Transmission: Autoinocculation, eye to eye, perinatal	Chronic sore eyes (up to 18 months if untreated) Profuse green discharge on waking Minimal itching	Inferior conjunctival follicles Superficial corneal neovascular area Pre-auricular LN ± Genitourinary signs (e.g. urethritis, cervicitis)	Neonatal conjunctivitis (Opthalmia neonatorum) is a notifiable disease and warrants urgent paediatric referral

Diagnosis	Background	Key symptoms	Key signs	Additional information
Subconjunctival haemorrhage	Common with increasing age Common causes: Idiopathic, trauma, cough/strain, systemic illness, hypertension Often recurrent Usually resolves within 2 wks	Sudden onset red eye No pain No eye discharge	Localised conjunctival haemorrhage Normal visual acuity ± High BP	Consider referral if history of trauma and posterior edge of haemorrhage not visible
Episcleritis	Inflammation of superficial sclera Benign Often self-limiting	Mild eye discomfort No discharge	Unilateral Diffuse red scleral patch Normal palpebral conjunctiva ± Inflammatory scleral nodule(s) near limbus	
Keratitis	Inflammation of the cornea Bacterial, fungal or viral cause Risk factors for bacterial keratitis: Contact lens wear, dry eyes, trauma, prolonged use of topical steroids	Severe gritty eye pain Blurred vision	Circumcorneal injection Hazy cornea Purulent discharge Photophobia Reduced visual acuity ± White/yellow level of pus in anterior chamber (hypopyon)	Urgent ophthalmology review due to risk of ulceration
Primary angle closure glaucoma (See Painful eye)				
Scleritis	Age 30–40 yrs ≈20% associated with connective tissue disease (e.g. RA)	Unilateral or bilateral involvement Deep intense eye pain Pain prevents sleep at night	Marked injection of the sclera Scleral swelling Visual disturbance Photophobia	Urgent referral as risk of perforation and/or visual loss
Kawasaki's disease	Commonest cause of acquired heart disease in UK children A systemic vasculitis Commonly ≤5 yrs age	Fever >5 days Irritable Red mouth and feet ± Atypical features (i.e. vomiting, swollen joints)	Fever >5 days Plus ≥4 of the following: Dry fissured lips or strawberry tongue Bilateral non-purulent conjunctivitis Polymorphous rash Oedema and erythema of palms/soles followed by desquamation of affected skin Tender cervical LN >1.5 cm	Urgent paediatric referral Common complications: Coronary artery aneurysms and MI

Watery eye

Diagnosis	Background	Key symptoms	Key signs	Additional information
Conjunctivitis (See Red eye)				
Foreign body (See Painful eye)				
Ectropion	Sagging and eversion of lower lid Loss of normal tear drainage Common in old age, owing to senile loss of orbital muscle and fat Other causes: Skin scarring, facial nerve palsy	Dry eyes	Unilateral or bilateral Everted lower-lid margin Injected conjunctivae	Secondary infection is common
Entropion	Inversion of lower lid Results in corneal irritation Associated with: Advancing age, scarring, ocular spasm	Gritty eye(s)	Unilateral or bilateral Inverted lower-lid margin Inturned eyelashes ± Red eye(s) ± Corneal abrasion	

Diagnosis	Background	Key symptoms	Key signs	Additional information
Congenital nasolacrimal duct obstruction	Common in infants aged <1 month Often spontaneously resolves in the first year of life	Persistent watery or sticky eye	Usually unilateral Normal sclera Normal conjunctivae Normal lid and lashes	Refer if persistent symptoms beyond 12 months
Dacryocystitis	Infection of the lacrimal sac Due to blockage of naso-lacrimal duct Commonly >40 yrs age or infants	Watery eye Pain over lacrimal sac	Unilateral Tender lump at medial canthus	Exclude pre-septal or orbital cellulitis Requires urgent antibiotics

Chapter 3
Ear, Nose and Throat

Blocked nose or rhinorrhoea

Diagnosis	Background	Key symptoms	Key signs	Additional information
Viral infection	Causes: rhinoviruses, RSV, Influenza, rotaviruses Usually self-limiting Droplet spread	Malaise ± Sore throat ± Cough ± Myalgia	Fever Normal respiratory examination ± Cervical LN	Complications include: Pneumonia, otitis media, tonsillitis
Allergic rhinitis	Seasonal or perennial symptoms Common allergens: Pollen, house dust mite, animal dander, occupational chemicals (e.g. flour) Family history of atopy	Symptoms within hours of exposure Itchy nose Sneezing Bilateral watery nasal discharge ± Itchy/watery eyes ± Nosebleeds	Bilateral swollen nasal turbinates ± Nasal polyps	
Vasomotor rhinitis	No history of allergy or URTI Can be precipitated by environmental factors: Cold weather, high humidity, cigarette smoke	Chronic nasal obstruction Bilateral watery nasal discharge Sneezing ± Nosebleeds	Bilateral swollen nasal turbinates ± Nasal polyps	Overuse of sympathomimetic vasoconstrictor nasal sprays can cause rebound chronic nasal congestion (Rhinitis medicamentosa)
Acute sinusitis (See Facial pain)				
Nasal polyp	Outgrowths of mucosa from nose and/or sinus cavity Commonly middle meatus Small polyps may be asymptomatic M>F Associated with: Chronic sinusitis, asthma and allergy Recurrence is common	Progressive nasal obstruction Watery nasal discharge Post-nasal drip Snoring ± Sleep apnoea	Usually bilateral Pale smooth grape-like swelling(s) Mobile Not sensitive to touch Reduced or absent sense of smell	A unilateral polyp requires ENT assessment to exclude malignancy Purulent nasal discharge suggests infection Refer routinely if polyps bilateral
Nasal septal deviation	Causes: Congenital or trauma Associated with recurrent sinusitis	Unilateral nasal blockage	Septum lies convex to one side Hypertrophied turbinates on opposite side of deviated septum	A bulging septum after recent nasal trauma may be a septal haematoma
Adenoid hyperplasia	Pre-pubescent children Adenoids normally atrophy by age ≤15 yrs Associated with recurrent middle ear infection/effusion and sinusitis	Mouth breathing often at night Daytime fatigue (due to lack of sleep) Otalgia Deafness ± Sleep apnoea	Evidence of recurrent URTI ± Enlarged tonsils	Persistent fatigue can cause problems at school Consider ENT referral

Differential Diagnosis in Primary Care, 1st edition. By Nairah Rasul and Mehmood Syed. © 2009 Blackwell Publishing, ISBN: 978-1-4051-8036-8

Diagnosis	Background	Key symptoms	Key signs	Additional information
Chronic sinusitis (Chronic rhinosinusitis)	Paranasal sinus inflammation Nose frequently involved Common pathogens: Anaerobes, gram-negative bacteria, *Staphylococcus aureus* Common risk factors: URTI, smoking, asthma, allergy, DM, swimming, dental infection	*≥1 of the following lasting >12 wks:* Facial pain/pressure Purulent nasal discharge Post-nasal drip Reduction/loss of smell ± Cough ± Bad breath (halitosis) ± Malaise ± Headache ± Upper toothache	Tenderness over sinuses Facial pain worse on stooping Normal respiratory examination ± Fever	Consider ENT referral

Dysphagia

Diagnosis	Background	Key symptoms	Key signs	Additional information
Cerebrovascular accident (Stroke)				
Subtypes:				
Ischaemic CVA	≈70% of all strokes Commonly >70 yrs age Risk factors: Hypertension, DM, AF, IHD, smoking, obesity, immobility, vasculitis, previous TIA, clotting disorder, hyperlipidaemia Symptom resolution within 24h indicates a TIA	Sudden or step-wise progression in neurological symptoms Occurs over hours/days ± Fall with or without LoC	Hypertension ± Confusion Focal or neurological signs, determined by area and severity of infarction	TIAs require urgent assessment due to further risk of stroke Exclude irregular heartbeat and carotid bruit
Subtypes of ischaemic CVA:				
Cerebral infarct			Dysphasia Contralateral hemiplegia/sensory deficit Homonymous hemianopia	
Brainstem infarct			Altered level of consciousness Ataxia Quadriplegia Cranial nerve defect	
Lacunar infarct			Normal conscious level Dysphasia Pure hemimotor deficit or Pure hemisensory deficit or Mixed motor/sensory deficit Unilateral limb ataxia	
Haemorrhagic CVA	Risk factors: Anticoagulants, head trauma, Berry aneurysm, hypertension, brain tumour	Acute onset severe headache Rapid progression of neurological symptoms	Focal or global depending on area and severity of haemorrhage, as above *If severe:* Meningism Coma	Emergency CT brain
Gastric carcinoma	Age >55 yrs M:F ratio: ≈3:1 Risk factors: Smoking, *H. pylori* infection, family history, atrophic gastritis, pernicious anaemia, blood group A High prevalence in Japan and China	New onset dyspepsia >4 wks Weight loss Vomiting Anorexia Abdominal pain	Anaemia Epigastric mass Palpable left supraclavicular LN (Virchow's node) Melaena	

Diagnosis	Background	Key symptoms	Key signs	Additional information
Benign oesophageal stricture	Chronic history of GORD Risk factors: Chronic ingestion of NSAIDs, iron, bisphosphonates, potassium preparations	Dyspepsia Difficulty swallowing solids Regurgitation ± Nocturnal cough	Normal examination	Weight loss or anaemia suggests malignancy
Oesophageal carcinoma	Commonly squamous cell or adenocarcinoma Age >60 yrs M:F ratio: ≈2:1 Risk factors: Smoking, alcoholic spirits, Barrett's oesophagus, achalsia, nitrosamine preserves	Progressive dysphagia Initially solids then liquids Weight loss Vomiting Anorexia	Cachexia Anaemia Cervical LN	
Motor neurone disease	Rapidly progressive Middle-age M:F ratio: ≈3:2	Slurred speech Nasal regurgitation Limb weakness Stumbling gait	*Bulbar palsy:* Dysarthria Nasal speech Absent gag reflex Fasciculating and weak tongue *LMN signs:* Muscle fasciculations Hyporeflexia *UMN signs:* Weakness of arm extensors and leg flexors Hyperreflexia Upgoing plantars No sensory, sphincter or oculomotor deficit	Dysphagia is often a late symptom
Myasthenia Gravis	Acquired condition Antibody mediated autoimmune disorder ≈15% associated with thymoma ≈75% associated with thymic hyperplasia Precipitating factors include: Pregnancy, infection, drugs	Muscular fatigue Common muscles involved: Extra-ocular muscles, limbs, bulbar and or respiratory	Asymmetrical diplopia or ptosis Rapid muscle fatigue on exercise Shoulder girdle weakness > pelvic girdle weakness Normal tone reflexes and sensation ± Facial weakness ± Dysarthria	Respiratory muscle involvement requires emergency airway management
Limited cutaneous systemic sclerosis (CREST syndrome)	Autoimmune connective tissue disease Age 30–40 yrs M<F	Fatigue Myalgia Swollen hands	*C*alcinosis: calcific hand nodules *R*aynaud's phenomenon: finger ischaemia o*E*sophageal dysmotility: dysphagia *S*clerodactyly: skin tightening of hands/feet *T*elangiectasia: generalised	Internal organs may be involved
Oesophageal achalasia	Incomplete relaxation of the lower oesophageal (cardiac) sphincter Onset 20–40 yrs age Associated with oesophageal carcinoma	Gradual onset over years Dysphagia of solids and liquids Regurgitation Retrosternal pain after meals Nocturnal cough	Normal examination	Chest infection may be precipitated by aspiration
Pharyngeal pouch	Age >70 yrs M:F ratio: ≈5:1	Regurgitation after meals Chronic cough	Halitosis Lump in neck (often left side) ± Chest infection (secondary to aspiration)	
Plummer Vinson syndrome	Formation of a post-cricoid oesophageal web Caused by iron deficiency Pre-malignant Typically middle-aged women	High dysphagia of solids Lethargy Weight loss	Anaemia Atrophic glossitis Angular stomatitis Kolionychia (spoon-shaped nails)	

Diagnosis	Background	Key symptoms	Key signs	Additional information
Quinsy	Peritonsillar abscess Often recent history of tonsillitis Commonly young adults	Unilateral pain in the throat Difficulty opening jaw (trismus) General malaise	Fever Drooling Ipsilateral tender cervical LN Peritonsillar oedema and exudate ± Erythematous enlarged tonsil	Emergency referral to ENT for incision and drainage

Earache

Diagnosis	Background	Key symptoms	Key signs	Additional information
Otitis media	Middle ear infection Common in children ≤5 yrs age Associated with URTI Often self-limiting within 3 days	Unilateral earache Ipsilateral deafness Malaise ± Purulent/bloody ear discharge (indicates TM perforation) ± Vomiting	Fever Pinna not tender Erythematous and bulging or perforated TM	Avoid topical aminoglycosides if perforated TM Hearing may take a few weeks to recover Consider ENT referral if otitis media in adults does not improve with antibiotics
Otitis externa	Inflammation of the external auditory canal Commonly middle-age Common causes: Primary infection, trauma, foreign body, impacted cerumen, allergy, psoriasis, seborrhoeic dermatitis	Unilateral earache Ipsilateral deafness Offensive ear discharge	Fever Inflammation and oedema of the external ear Ear discharge Debris in the ear canal Normal TM Traction on the pinna/tragus is painful Post-auricular LN	Consider ENT referral for microsuction if debris prevents effective topical treatment
Boil (Furuncle)	Deep infection of a hair follicle Affects external ear Usually *Staphlococcus aureus*	Severe earache ± Deafness (if meatus occluded)	Red swelling in the external ear canal Traction on the pinna/tragus is painful	Consider referral to ENT for i.v. antibiotics and wick insertion if treatment with oral antibiotics is unsuccessful
Referred pain	Common sources: Tonsillitis, pharyngitis, dental abscess, impacted molar	Vary depending on origin of pain	Normal ear examination	
Temporomandibular joint dysfunction	Abnormal jaw function Jaw anatomy may be normal or abnormal Onset early adolescence or adulthood Can persist into middle-age M:F ratio ≈1:4 Associated with bruxism and/or joint disease (e.g. arthritis)	Facial pain Headache Painful jaw	Crepitus on jaw movement Restricted jaw movement Painful jaw movement ± Depression or anxiety	
Mastoiditis	Complication of otitis media Acute or chronic infection Commonly young children Risk factor: Cholesteatoma	Progressive earache Pain felt behind the ear Irritable or crying infant	Fever Post-auricular swelling and erythema Tender mastoid ± Ear pushed forward ± Erythematous and bulging TM	Signs can be subtle in chronic mastoiditis so refer if suspicious Complications include cranial nerve palsies
Ramsay Hunt syndrome (Herpes zoster oticus)	Herpes zoster infection of VII nerve Causes an LMN facial nerve palsy Occasionally acoustic nerve is also affected	Severe deep pain in the ear Precedes onset of ear rash Vertigo Tinnitus	Yellow crops of vesicles on the pinna, TM and/or soft palate *Ipsilateral LMN facial palsy:* Facial droop Facial muscle weakness Loss of taste of anterior $^2/_3$ tongue Hyperacusis or Ipsilateral sensorineural deafness	

Epistaxis

Diagnosis	Background	Key symptoms	Key signs	Additional information
Trauma	Recent history: Nasal injury, nose picking, blowing nose, foreign body Epistaxis can be precipitated by use of topical nasal steroids or nasal infection	Epistaxis ± Pain	Bleeding often originates from Little's area of the septum	Consider cocaine abuse if septum appears atrophic
Rhinitis (See Blocked nose or rhinorrhoea)				
Thrombocytopenia				
Common subtypes:				
Idiopathic	IgG antibodies destroy platelets In children M = F Often self-limiting in children following viral infection Can become chronic in young adults M:F ratio ≈1:3	Often acute onset Prolonged, excessive or recurrent epistaxis Bleeding gums Spontaneous bruising ± Haemoptysis ± Haematemesis ± Blood in stool	Generalised petechiae Bruises	Splenomegaly or lymphadenopathy suggest a more sinister cause (e.g. marrow failure)
Alloimmune	History of blood transfusion Occurs 10 days to several months post-transfusion	As above	As above	
Drug induced	Drugs include: Warfarin, ibuprofen, carbamezapine, amiodarone, cimetidine, ranitidine, phenytoin, heparin, alcohol	As above	As above	
Nasopharygeal carcinoma	Poorly differentiated tumour Often occurs around the ostium of the Eustachian tube Prevalent in Chinese Risk factor: Tobacco use	Nasal obstruction Unilateral hearing loss Post-nasal discharge	Cervical LN Reduced smell (hyposmia) Ipsilateral deafness	

Conductive hearing loss*

Diagnosis	Background	Key symptoms	Key signs	Additional information
Impacted ear wax	Commonly elderly Risk factors: Hearing aids, cotton buds	Discomfort in the affected ear ± Tinnitus	Hard wax in the ear canal	
Middle ear effusion **(Glue ear)**	No active inflammation of the TM Children 4–7 yrs age M>F Associated with a blocked Eustachian tube (e.g. URTI, adenoid hypertrophy) Usually resolves within 3 months	Poor speech and language development Behavioural problems ± Earache	*Tympanic membrane:* Concave and opacified Dull with loss of light reflex Fluid level or bubbles behind TM	Developmental problems warrant an ENT referral Adults should be investigated to exclude nasopharyngeal carcinoma
Eustachian tube dysfunction	Blocked or impaired opening of ET Associated with: URTI, air travel, allergy Deafness may linger for weeks post-infection	Muffled hearing Sensation of fullness in the ear Dizziness or vertigo ± Earache	Normal auroscopy	

*Conductive hearing loss: *Weber's test:* Tuning fork is louder in the affected ear. *Rinne's test:* Bone conduction > air conduction on the affected side.

Diagnosis	Background	Key symptoms	Key signs	Additional information
Otosclerosis	Progressive sclerosis and ankylosis of the stapes to the oval window Autosomal dominant Presents 15–45 yrs age Sensorineural deafness also occurs if cochlea affected	Progressive hearing loss involves low frequencies Tinnitus ± Positional vertigo	Typically bilateral Normal auroscopy Bilateral conductive hearing loss ± Sensorineural loss ± Schwartze sign (pink TM, indicates bony vascularisation)	
Chronic suppurative otitis media	Symptoms are present ≥6 months: Chronic middle ear inflammation Chronic ear discharge TM perforation ± Active infection Risk factors: Recurrent otitis media, crowded housing, cranial facial anomalies (e.g. cleft palate)	Chronic ear discharge for ≥6 months Ear discomfort	Ear discharge (purulent/serous/ caseated) Granulation of middle ear ± Oedematous or polypoid middle ear mucosa Central perforation of TM	Beware attic/marginal TM perforation which may indicate a cholesteatoma
Otitis media	Middle ear infection Common in children ≤5 yrs age Associated with URTI Often self-limiting within 3 days	Unilateral earache Ipsilateral deafness Malaise ± Purulent/bloody ear discharge (indicates TM perforation) ± Vomiting	Fever Pinna not tender Erythematous and bulging or perforated TM	Avoid topical aminoglycosides if perforated TM Hearing may take a few weeks to recover Consider ENT referral if otitis media in adults does not improve with antibiotics
Otitis externa	Inflammation of the external auditory canal Commonly middle-age Common causes: Primary infection, trauma, foreign body, impacted cerumen, allergy, psoriasis, seborrhoeic dermatitis	Unilateral earache Ipsilateral deafness Offensive ear discharge	Fever Inflammation and oedema of the external ear Ear discharge Debris in the ear canal Normal TM Traction on the pinna/tragus is painful Post-auricular LN	Consider ENT referral for microsuction if debris prevents effective topical treatment
Nasal polyp (See Blocked nose or rhinorrhoea)				
Cholesteatoma	Growth of stratified squamous epithelium in the middle ear Can be locally invasive and erosive Commonly acquired Rarely congenital Risk factor: Ear trauma	Progressive unilateral hearing loss Painless Purulent ear discharge	Offensive ear discharge Flaky white debris in middle cleft Attic or marginal perforation of TM	Local expansion can result in vertigo, facial nerve palsy and/ or cerebral abscess

Sensorineural hearing loss*

Diagnosis	Background	Key symptoms	Key signs	Additional information
Presbyacusis	Progressive age-related hearing loss Loss in perception of high frequencies Age >60 yrs Risk factors: Noise pollution, family history, smoking, DM, hypertension	Progressive difficulty in understanding speech, especially in noisy environments ± Tinnitus	Bilateral hearing loss Normal auroscopy	Can lead to social isolation and depression and/or worsen cognitive impairment TM may become opacified with age
Paget's disease of the bone	Abnormal osteoclast activity Disorganised bone remodelling Results in larger and weaker bones Age >40 yrs M>F Commonly affects spine, skull and long bones ≈1% cases develop sarcoma	Often asymptomatic or Dull bony pain (e.g. backache) Worse on weight-bearing Progressive bone deformity Deafness	Bowing of tibia, femur and/or forearm Frontal bossing Deafness (CN VIII compression) Pathological fractures (e.g. femur)	

*Sensorineural hearing loss: *Weber's Test:*Tuning fork is louder in the normal ear. *Rinne's test:* Air conduction > bone conduction in both ears.

Diagnosis	Background	Key symptoms	Key signs	Additional information
Ménière's disease	Disorder of inner ear Age 20–50 yrs	Initially unilateral symptoms *Episodic attacks of:* Rotatory vertigo >20 mins Hearing loss (often low frequency) Tinnitus ± "fullness" in the ear Often full recovery between attacks	Normal auroscopy Nystagmus and nausea during acute attack	
Ototoxic medication	Irreversible or reversible vestibular or cochlear toxicity Common ototoxic drugs: Aminoglycosides, loop diuretics, aspirin Precipitated by impaired renal excretion	Tinnitus Gradual hearing loss ± Vertigo	Normal auroscopy	Vestibular effects may not be apparent in immobile patients
Acoustic neuroma	Tumour of the VIII (acoustic) nerve Typically benign and slow growing ≈95% cases are unilateral ≈5% cases are bilateral and associated with neurofibromatosis type 2	Gradual onset Hearing loss over months/years Tinnitus Ipsilateral occipital pain Mild vertigo	Unilateral sensorineural hearing loss Ipsilateral trigeminal nerve (V) palsy ± Ipsilateral cerebellar signs (advanced disease)	

Hoarse voice

Diagnosis	Background	Key symptoms	Key signs	Additional information
Acute laryngitis	Often viral Other causes: Sinusitis, smoking, excessive use of voice, post-intubation Self-limiting within 2 wks	Malaise Pain on using voice	Hoarse voice Normal throat examination	
Vocal cord nodules	Swellings of the true vocal cord Benign Associated with excessive use of voice Subsides within 48 h of voice rest	Vocal fatigue Loss in vocal range	Normal throat examination	
Aquired hypothyroidism	Age <60 yrs M<F Causes: Autoimmune, thyroiditis, TSH deficiency, postpartum, thyroidectomy, neck radiation, iodine deficiency, drugs (e.g. amiodarone, carbizamole) Associated with high cholesterol/ triglycerides and anaemia	Lethargy Weight gain Constipation Low mood Cold intolerance Menorrhagia	Deep hoarse voice Slow cognition (e.g. poor memory) Dry coarse skin Thinning hair Bradycardia Slow-relaxing tendon reflexes ± Goitre	Beware myxoedema in the elderly: Puffy eyes, hands and feet Cerebellar ataxia Hypothermia Seizures ± Coma
Gastro-oesophageal reflux disease (See Chest pain)				
Conversion disorder (Hysteria)	An alteration or loss of physical functioning in the absence of pathology Commonly triggered by repressed anxiety/stress Affects voluntary muscles	Acute onset hoarseness or aphonia	Normal swallow, gag and cough ± La belle difference (little concern regarding symptoms)	The sick role attracts attention, thus reducing any immediate emotional stress (Primary gain)
Laryngeal carcinoma	Commonly squamous cell Age >50 yrs M>F Risk factors: Smoking and alcohol	Persistent hoarseness Chronic cough ± Dysphagia ± Sore throat	Cervical LN Stridor (late sign)	Hoarseness >4 wks requires ENT referral to exclude malignancy

Diagnosis	Background	Key symptoms	Key signs	Additional information
Recurrent laryngeal nerve palsy	Causes include: Mediastinal carcinoma, aortic aneurysm, post-influenza, thyroid surgery	Change in quality of voice	Bovine (unexplosive) cough	

Mouth ulcers

Diagnosis	Background	Key symptoms	Key signs	Additional information
Trauma	Mechanical, chemical or thermal History indicates the cause (e.g. bitten tongue, bleaching of dentures, hot beverages)	Localised sore in the mouth	Often shallow ulcers with non-raised margins	
Recurrent aphthous ulceration (Aphthous stomatitis)	Onset common in childhood Less common with advancing age Non-contagious Causes include: Idiopathic, familial, stress			Exclude iron/vitamin B12/folate deficiency
Subtypes:				
Minor ulcers	Commonest type Resolve within 7–10 days Heals without scarring	Mild pain ± Prodromal tingling	Ulcers <1 cm diameter Usually multiple Yellow/grey round ulcers Erythematous halo around ulcer	
Major ulcers	Resolve within 2 wks to several months Heals with scarring	Very painful ulcers ± Prodromal tingling	Ulcers >1 cm diameter Usually solitary Yellow/grey round ulcer Erythematous halo around ulcer	Suspect malignancy if the ulcer is solitary, unresolving and painless
Pinpoint ulcers ("Herpetiform" ulcers)	Resolves within 1 wk to 2 months Not Herpes related	Mild pain ± Prodromal tingling	Ulcers 0.1–0.2 cm diameter Usually multiple May coalesce	
Oral candidiasis (Oral thrush)	Overgrowth of commensal *Candida* Common in babies Risk factors: Antibiotics, dentures, dummies, steroid inhalers, immunosupression, iron/folate deficiency	Painful mouth	White coalesced plaques Underlying inflamed friable mucosa Angular stomatitis	
Acute necrotising ulcerative gingivitis (Vincent's infection)	Bacterial gum infection Caused by poor oral hygiene	Malaise Painful and bleeding gums Foul metallic taste	Fever Halitosis Cervical LN Punched out ragged gingival ulcers	There is concomitant pharyngeal inflammation in Vincent's angina
Oral herpes simplex virus (Cold sores)	Acute viral infection Typically due to HSV Type I			
Subtypes:				
Primary HSV	First episode of infection Common in pre-school children Spread by saliva Incubation 3–10 days Post-recovery, virus remains dormant in the sensory ganglia	Often asymptomatic or *Acute herpetic gingivostomatitis*: Painful mouth ulcers Bleeding gums	*Acute herpetic gingivostomatitis*: Fever Dehydration Cervical LN Ulceration of tongue, palate and buccal mucosa Multiple coalescing oral vesicles	
Recurrent HSV	HSV re-activation Trigger factors: Immunosupression, stress, sun exposure, menstruation Highly contagious Spread by saliva Spontaneous healing over 1–2 wks No scarring	Facial tingling and itching Followed by vesicle eruption within hours/days	Multiple weeping vesicles around mouth and nares Vesicles crust before healing	

Diagnosis	Background	Key symptoms	Key signs	Additional information
Hand, foot and mouth disease	Caused by Coxsackie enterovirus Commonly <5 yrs age Spread by faecal–oral route Self-limiting within 1 wk	Malaise Anorexia Followed by mouth ulcers and then skin lesions ± Pruritis	Mild fever *Mouth lesions:* Multiple yellow ulcers Surrounded by erythematous halo *Hand and foot lesions:* Erythematous macules become grey vesicles on erythematous base *Skin rash:* Erythematous maculopapular rash	NOT related to cattle "Foot and mouth" disease
Coeliac disease (See Diarrhoea)				
Inflammatory bowel disease (See Diarrhoea)				
Oral carcinoma	Commonly squamous cell Often malignant Elderly ≈50% affect the tongue Risk factors: Alcoholic spirits and tobacco	A persistent slow-growing ulcer Associated bleeding Halitosis	Submandibular and cervical LN Unresolving ulcer ± White patch (leukoplakia) ± Red patch (erythroplakia)	Refer for biopsy
Erythema multiforme	Age <40 yrs Trigger factors include: HSV, hepatitis, *Streptococcus*, radiotherapy Often mild Usually self-limiting within 3 wks	Acute onset symptoms Non-tender skin rash Affects: Mouth, genitals, palms, soles, extensor surfaces of arms and legs	*Target lesions:* Round macular erythematous lesions Purplish centre with pale outer ring Symmetrical peripheral distribution Spreads centrally ± Blistering of lesions	Stevens-Johnsons syndrome: A severe drug-induced form involving the mucous membranes
Bechet's disease	Multi-system autoimmune disorder Age 15–45 yrs M>F Associated with HLA-B51	Recurrent symptoms Fatigue Painful mouth and genital ulcers Tender shins Painful eye	Fever Oral and genital ulcers with scarring Erythema nodosum Anterior uveitis ± Symptomatic involvement of other systems (e.g DVT, diarrhoea, arthralgia)	
Syphilitic chancre (See Vulval ulcers)				

Vertigo

Diagnosis	Background	Key symptoms	Key signs	Additional information
Viral vestibular neuronitis and labyrinthitis	Often recent history of URTI Usually resolves within 4 wks Mild unsteadiness can persist for months	Acute onset vertigo Worse on general movement Nausea/vomiting	Unsteady gait Nystagmus (horizontal or rotatory) Normal auroscopy No deafness or tinnitus No neurological deficit	Risk of benign positional vertigo after vestibular neuronitis
Vertebrobasilar insufficiency	Commonly due to atherosclerosis of vertebral arteries Associated with ≈20% of all strokes M>F Risk factors: Advancing age, smoking, DM, hypertension, IHD, obesity, temporal arteritis	Gradual onset vertigo Intermittent episodes ± Worse on turning head Headache Visual disturbance (e.g. double vision) Unsteady gait	Focal neurology varies according to the site of ischaemia *Common signs:* Altered consciousness Visual field defect Oculomotor palsy Gait ataxia Contralateral hemiparesis	Vertigo is common and may be the only symptom

Diagnosis	Background	Key symptoms	Key signs	Additional information

Ménière's Disease	Disorder of inner ear
	Age 20–50 yrs
		Initially unilateral symptoms
		Episodic attacks of:
		Rotatory vertigo >20 mins
		Hearing loss (often low
		  frequency)
		Tinnitus ± "fullness" in the ear
		Often full recovery between
		  attacks
			Normal auroscopy
			Nystagmus and nausea during
			  acute attack	

Benign positional vertigo	Displacement of otoconia (debris)
	  within the vestibular labyrinth
	M:F ratio: ≈1:2
	Common after head injury or
	  vestibular neuronitis
	Often resolves spontaneously
	  within months
		Head turning provokes vertigo
		Lasts a few seconds/minutes
		No vomiting
			Positive Hallpike Manoeuvre
			Normal auroscopy	

Eustachian tube dysfunction	Blocked or impaired opening
	  of ET
	Associated with: URTI, air travel,
	  allergy
	Deafness may linger for weeks
	  post-infection
		Muffled hearing
		Sensation of fullness in the ear
		Dizziness or vertigo
		± Earache
			Normal auroscopy	

Ototoxic medication (See Sensorineural deafness)				

Acoustic neuroma	Tumour of the VIII (acoustic)
	  nerve
	Typically benign and slow
	  growing
	≈95% cases are unilateral
	≈5% cases are bilateral
	  and associated with
	  neurofibromatosis type 2
		Gradual onset symptoms
		Hearing loss over months/years
		Tinnitus
		Ipsilateral occipital pain
		Mild vertigo
			Unilateral sensorineural hearing
			  loss
			Ipsilateral trigeminal nerve (V)
			  palsy
			± Ipsilateral cerebellar signs
			  (advanced disease)	

Ramsay Hunt syndrome
(Herpes zoster oticus)
	Herpes zoster infection of VII
	  nerve
	Causes a LMN facial nerve palsy
	Occasionally acoustic nerve is also
	  affected
		Severe deep pain in the ear
		Precedes onset of ear rash
		Vertigo
		Tinnitus
			Yellow crops of vesicles on the
			  pinna, TM and/or soft palate
			Ipsilateral LMN facial palsy:
			Facial droop
			Facial muscle weakness
			Loss of taste of anterior
			  $^2/_3$ tongue
			Hyperacusis or
			Ipsilateral sensorineural deafness	

Subclavian steal syndrome	Stenosis of subclavian artery
	  proximal to vertebral artery
	Retrograde blood flow from
	  vertebrobasilar circulation to
	  subclavian artery
	Affects left artery > right artery
	Often due to atherosclerosis
	May resolve spontaneously due
	  to collateral formation
		Symptoms worse on exercising
		  affected arm:
		Vertigo
		Unilateral or bilateral visual loss
		Transient dysarthria
		Paraesthesia of face
		Pulsatile tinnitus
		Falls ± LoC
			Signs reproduced on exercising
			  affected arm:
			Transient gait ataxia
			Transient diplopia
			Reduced BP >20 mmHg in
			  affected arm
			± Transient hemiparesis
			± Reduced/absent arm pulses	

Chapter 4
Thorax

Acute breathlessness

Diagnosis	Background	Key symptoms	Key signs	Additional information
Bronchiolitis	Usually due to Respiratory Syncytial Virus Age <1 yr Common in winter Droplet spread Self-limiting	Coryzal symptoms Poor feeding Shortness of breath Cough	Hyperinflated chest Tachypnoea >50 breaths/min Tachycardia >160 bpm Hyper-resonant chest percussion Widespread fine crackles Wheeze	Dehydration or respiratory distress warrants an emergency admission
Acute exacerbation of asthma	Reversible airways obstruction Almost daily PEFR variability ≥20% PEFR improves ≥20% with beta agonist Precipitated by: Cold air, infection, exercise, emotion, allergens, drugs	Shortness of breath Chest tightness Nocturnal cough Wheeze worse on waking	Tachypnoea Tachycardia Hyperinflated chest Widespread polyphonic wheeze Prolonged expiration ± Reduced air entry ± Difficulty completing sentences	Admit if severe attack
Acute exacerbation of COPD	History of stable COPD Often history of smoking Common in winter Exacerbated by: Infection, environmental pollutants ≈30% have no identifiable cause	Increasing breathlessness over days Chest tightness Cough and increased sputum Reduced exercise tolerance	Tachypnoea Hyperinflated chest Cough and sputum (± purulent) Coarse crackles Bilateral wheeze	Consider admission if: Severe dehydration Confusion and/or cyanosis New onset peripheral oedema Respiratory distress
Croup (Acute laryngotracheitis)	Usually a viral infection Affects larynx and trachea Commonly children aged 1–3 yrs Autumn and spring epidemics Self-limiting	Cough Coryzal symptoms Noisy breathing Symptoms worse at night ± Shortness of breath	Barking cough Stridor Hoarse cry/voice ± Intercostal recession ± Tachypnoea	
Acute left ventricular failure	Causes: IHD, cardiomyopathy, hypertension, mitral regurgitation, aortic stenosis, arrhythmia, PHT, fluid overload, alcohol abuse, hyperthyroidism, Paget's, anaemia	Breathless on exertion Orthopnoea PND Nocturnal cough Weight loss Fatigue ± Frothy pink sputum ± Haemoptysis	Tachypnoea Tachycardia Hypotension Displaced apex S3 (Gallop rhythm) Bibasal end-inspiratory crackles Wheeze (cardiac asthma) ± Cyanosis	Consider admission
Generalised anxiety disorder (See Anxiety or Insomnia)				
Pneumonia (See Cough)				

Differential Diagnosis in Primary Care, 1st edition. By Nairah Rasul and Mehmood Syed. Published 2009 by Blackwell Publishing, ISBN: 978-1-4051-8036-8

Diagnosis	Background	Key symptoms	Key signs	Additional information
Anaphylaxis	Allergens include: Pulses, nuts, fish, shellfish, eggs, milk, insect stings, drugs, latex	Typically acute onset Chest tightness Pruritis Runny nose Palpitations Nausea and vomiting	Tachycardia Hypotension Generalised urticaria and erythema Stridor Angio-oedema Tongue swelling ± Wheeze	Itchy palate or ear suggests airway involvement If shocked DO NOT delay i.m. adrenaline
Pneumothorax	Common causes: Trauma, spontaneous, pre-existing lung disease, iatrogenic Risk factors: Smoking, subpleural bleb/bullae, tall thin stature Recurrence is common	Pleuritic chest pain	*On affected side:* Reduced chest expansion Reduced air entry Hyper-resonant to percussion	Small pneumothoraces may be asymptomatic A deviated trachea away from the affected side indicates a tension pneumothorax
Pulmonary embolism	Commonly a venous thrombus Risk factors: Immobility, recent surgery, pregnancy, puerperium, malignancy, family history, COCP, HRT, thrombophilia, smoking, obesity	Pleuritic chest pain ± Haemoptysis ± Dizziness ± Syncope	Fever Tachycardia Tachypnoea Hypotension Raised JVP Pleural rub ± Swollen calf (suggests DVT)	Recurrent emboli may cause chronic breathlessness
Pleural effusion	Common causes: Malignancy, infection, PE, cardiac failure, hypoproteinaemia, hypothyroidism, inflammation (e.g. RA, SLE)	Pleuritic chest pain Breathless on exertion	*On affected side:* Reduced chest expansion "Stony" dullness to percussion Reduced air entry Bronchial breathing above effusion	
Diabetic ketoacidosis (See Upper abdominal pain)				
Churg-Strauss syndrome	Generalised systemic vasculitis Affects small to medium arteries/veins Associated with asthma, allergic rhinitis and eosinophilia Vasculitis presents years after onset asthma	Fatigue Weight loss Arthralgia Myalgia Runny nose Worsening asthma Haemoptysis	Vary according to organ involvement *Common signs:* Fever Skin purpura and nodules Peripheral neuropathy ≥2 nerves (Mononeuritis multiplex) Severe asthma Heart failure	

Chronic breathlessness

Diagnosis	Background	Key symptoms	Key signs	Additional information
Obesity	BMI >30 kg/m² Common risk factors: Family history, inactivity, diet, social deprivation, alcohol abuse Associated with: IHD, hypertension, Type II DM, sleep apnoea, endometrial carcinoma, infertility, osteoarthritis, increased oestrogen	Weight gain may be rapid or gradual Breathless on exertion	BMI >30 kg/m² Pseudogynaecomastia Normal respiratory examination	
Chronic obstructive pulmonary disease (Chronic bronchitis or emphysema)	Progressive airways obstruction Little or no reversibility FEV1 <80% predicted FEV1/FVC <70% Age >40 yrs Causes: Smoking, occupational pollutants, alpha-1 anti-trypsin deficiency	Cough and sputum on most days Lasts ≥3 months over 2 successive years Breathless on exertion ± Weight loss	Tachypnoea Hyperinflated chest Reduced chest expansion Quiet breath sounds Wheeze Resonant on percussion ± Accessory muscle use ± Cyanosis ± Flapping tremor	

Diagnosis	Background	Key symptoms	Key signs	Additional information
Cardiac failure	Due to low or high cardiac output Causes of low-output failure: IHD, cardiomyopathy, hypertension, mitral regurgitation, aortic stenosis, arrhythmia, PHT, fluid overload, alcohol abuse Causes of *high-output failure*: Hyperthyroidism, Paget's, anaemia			
Subtypes:				
Left ventricular failure	Causes: IHD, cardiomyopathy, hypertension, mitral regurgitation, aortic stenosis, arrhythmia, PHT, fluid overload, alcohol abuse, hyperthyroidism, Paget's, anaemia	Breathless on exertion Orthopnoea PND Nocturnal cough Weight loss Fatigue ± Frothy pink sputum ± Haemoptysis	Tachypnoea Tachycardia Hypotension Displaced apex S3 (Gallop rhythm) Bibasal end-inspiratory crackles Wheeze (cardiac asthma) ± Cyanosis	Consider admission if acute
Right ventricular failure	Common causes: LVF and chronic lung disease	Breathless on exertion Leg and abdominal swelling Nausea Anorexia Fatigue	Raised JVP Leg and sacral pitting oedema Ascites Hepatomegaly (may be pulsatile) ± Mild jaundice ± Cyanosis	
Asthma	Reversible airways obstruction Almost daily PEFR variability ≥20% PEFR improves ≥20% with beta agonist Precipitated by: Cold air, infection, exercise, emotion, allergens, drugs	Intermittent breathlessness Chest tightness Wheeze Worse on waking Nocturnal cough	Hyperinflated chest Widespread polyphonic wheeze Prolonged expiration	Admit if severe attack
Anaemia			Vary depending on underlying cause	
Subtypes:				
Microcytic anaemia	MCV <76 fl Often due to iron deficiency Causes: Chronic blood loss, poor diet, pregnancy, malabsorption	Breathless on exertion Fatigue Palpitations Chest pain	Pallor Kolionychia (spoon-shaped nails) Pale nails Glossitis Angular stomatitis	
Normocytic anaemia	MCV 76–96 fl Often due to haemolysis or chronic disease Causes include: Genetic (e.g. spherocytosis, sickle cell) or acquired (e.g. immune, malaria)	As above	Pallor Jaundice Hepatosplenomegaly	
Macrocytic anaemia	MCV >96 fl Often due to folate or vitamin B12 deficiency Causes: Poor diet (e.g. alcoholic), pernicious anaemia, malabsorption, malignancy, pregnancy, hypothyroidism, drugs (e.g. anticonvulsants, methotrexate)	As above	Pallor Glossitis Aphthous mouth ulcers	

Diagnosis	Background	Key symptoms	Key signs	Additional information

Lung carcinoma (Bronchial carcinoma)	Incidence increases >40 yrs age
	Risk factors: Smoking, industrial pollutants (e.g. arsenic, iron oxide, asbestos), radiation
		Chronic cough
		Haemoptysis
		Chest or shoulder pain
		Weight loss
			Cachexia
			Anaemia
			Clubbing
			Supraclavicular or axillary LN
			Gynaecomastia
			± Chest signs
			  (e.g. consolidation, effusion)
			± Metastases
			  (e.g. bony tenderness,
			  confusion, hepatomegaly)
				Histological subtypes:
				Squamous ≈30%
				Adenocarcinoma ≈30%
				Small (oat cell) ≈25%
				Large cell ≈15%
				Alveolar cell <1%

Bronchiectasis	Chest infection leads to permanently dilated bronchi/ bronchioles Usual onset in adulthood Common causes: Post-infective, RA, bronchial obstruction, hypogammaglobulinaemia, congenital (e.g. cystic fibrosis)	Chronic daily cough Duration months to years Copious purulent sputum Haemoptysis Malaise Pleuritic chest pain	Fever Coarse inspiratory crackles Wheeze ± Clubbing (severe disease)	
Dilated cardiomyopathy (Congestive cardiomyopathy)	Commonest cardiomyopathy Dilatation and reduced contractility of left ± right ventricle Age 20–60 yrs M>F Causes: Idiopathic, familial, alcohol abuse, viral, thyrotoxicosis, cocaine abuse, haemochromatosis, autoimmune, hypertension, IHD	Fatigue Progressive exercise intolerance	Tachypnoea Tachycardia Hypotension Raised JVP Displaced apex S3 (Gallop rhythm) Wheeze (cardiac asthma) Bibasal end-inspiratory crackles Leg and sacral pitting oedema Ascites Hepatomegaly (may be pulsatile) ± Cyanosis	Ventricular arrhythmias can cause sudden death
Recurrent pulmonary emboli (see Acute breathlessness)				
Aortic stenosis	Causes: Senile calcification, congenital Results in LVH This can progress to CCF Associated with bacterial endocarditis and sudden death	*Symptoms worse on exertion:* Shortness of breath Angina ± Dizziness or syncope	Slow rising pulse Small volume pulse Narrow pulse pressure Palpable LV heave Palpable systolic thrill S2 soft or absent Ejection systolic murmur Loudest at aortic area and left sternal edge Radiates to apex and carotids	Aortic sclerosis sounds similar but is distingushed from AS by: Normal pulse Normal S2 No radiation to carotids Absent systolic thrill
Fibrosing alveolitis	Restrictive interstitial lung disease Characterised by alveolar inflammation and fibrosis Onset late middle-age M:F ratio: ≈2:1 Risk factors: Exposure to silica, asbestos, heavy metals, mouldy foliage	Coryzal symptoms Persistent dry cough Progressive exercise intolerance Weight loss Arthralgia Myalgia	Tachypnoea Central cyanosis Clubbing Fine bibasal end-inspiratory crackles	

Diagnosis	Background	Key symptoms	Key signs	Additional information
Sarcoidosis	Chronic multisystem disorder Characterised by epithelioid non-caseating granulomata Typical onset 20–40 yrs age Most frequent and severe in Afro-Carribeans $\approx^2/_3$ cases resolve $\approx^1/_3$ become chronic with relapses and remissions	Vary or may be asymptomatic *Non-specific symptoms:* Fever Fatigue Weight loss *Pulmonary symptoms include:* Dry cough Progressive exertional dyspnoea Chest pain *Extrapulmonary symptoms include:* Red rash Blurred vision Dry eyes Arthralgia	*Common signs:* Generalised maculopapular rash Erythema nodosum Lupus pernio (violaceous swelling of nose/cheeks) Posterior uveitis Cranial nerve palsy (e.g. Bell's palsy)	Lupus pernio is pathognomonic
Extrinsic allergic alveolitis	Pneumonitis triggered by inhalation of allergens in sensitised individuals Common allergens: Fungal spores and avian proteins Risk factors: Farming, keeping birds, hot tubs	Symptoms can be acute or chronic *Acute symptoms <12 h from exposure:* Rigors Myalgia Chest tightness Dry cough *Chronic symptoms:* Progressive exertional dyspnoea Weight loss	Signs can be acute or chronic *Acute symptoms <12 h from exposure:* Fever Few scattered crackles at bases *Chronic signs:* Cyanosis Right ventricular failure ± Clubbing	
Occupational lung disease	Any lung disease caused directly by the work environment Develops months/years post-exposure Common diseases: Occupational asthma, asbestosis, coal worker's pneumoconiosis, byssinosis, COPD	Vary depending on underlying allergen *Common symptoms:* Progessive breathlessness Chest tightness Symptoms improve away from work	Vary depending on underlying allergen and length of exposure *Common signs:* Poor PEFR Wheeze Reduced air entry	Consider referral to a respiratory specialist for confirmation of diagnosis

Chest Pain

Diagnosis	Background	Key symptoms	Key signs	Additional information
Gastro-oesophageal reflux disease	Risk factors: Obesity, smoking, alcohol, caffeine, tight clothes, big meals, pregnancy, drugs (e.g. TCA, NSAID), hiatus hernia, surgery in achalasia	Retrosternal burning pain Worse on stooping, lying or eating Relieved by antacids Water/acid brash Belching Nocturnal wheeze or cough	Normal abdominal examination Normal cardiorespiratory examination ± Hoarse voice	Refer for urgent upper GI endoscopy if: >55 yrs and persistent symptoms >4 wks Or at any age if: Weight loss Dysphagia Anaemia Vomiting
Generalised anxiety disorder (See Anxiety)				
Musculoskeletal injury	History of muscle/rib trauma or strain	Localised chest pain Worse on movement Pain on deep inspiration	Normal cardiorespiratory examination Focal chest wall tenderness	
Costochondritis	Idiopathic inflammation of the costal cartilage Commonly affects second costochondral junction Usually self-limiting	Localised chest pain Worse on sneezing, coughing and movement	Unilateral Focal tenderness on palpation ± Costocartilage swelling (Tietze's syndrome)	
Pleurisy	Pleural inflammation Causes: Viral/bacterial infection, PE, pneumothorax, effusion	Pleuritic chest pain Localised pain	Chest wall non-tender on palpation Pleural rub	

Diagnosis	Background	Key symptoms	Key signs	Additional information
Ischaemic heart disease	M>F Risk factors: Advancing age, family history, South Asian, obesity, hyperlipidaemia, DM, smoking, hypertension			
Presentations:				
Stable angina	Stable exercise tolerance	Central heavy crushing chest pain or epigastric pain ± Radiation to neck, jaw, arm(s) Worse on exertion, cold, emotion, eating Duration <20 mins Relieved by rest ± Relieved by GTN	Signs often absent	Other causes of stable angina include: Tachyarrhythmia, aortic stenosis, arteritis, HOCM, anaemia
Acute coronary syndrome				Requires emergency admission
Subtypes of ACS:				
Unstable angina	Worsening exercise tolerance ± History of stable angina	Central heavy crushing chest pain or epigastric pain ± Radiation to neck, jaw, arm(s) Occurs on minimal exertion/ at rest Duration <20 mins ± Relieved by GTN	Signs often absent	
Myocardial infarction		Acute onset Central heavy crushing chest pain or epigastric pain ± Radiation to neck, jaw, arm(s) Duration >20 mins Not relieved by rest or GTN Nausea Sweating Shortness of breath ± Collapse	Low-grade fever <39°C Anxiety Cold and clammy Systolic murmur ± Heart failure ± Loss of consciousness	Beware of silent MI in the elderly or diabetic. Symptoms are often atypical
Shingles (Herpes zoster) (For Ophthalmic shingles see Painful eye)	Reactivation of varicella zoster History of chicken pox Common in elderly and immunosuppressed Severity increases with age	Malaise Burning, painful or itchy skin Followed by onset of rash	Fever Onset of rash 1 to 3 days after pain Vesicular rash on an erythematous base Vesicles crust and dry over the following 2 wks Usually one dermatome affected Rash does not cross the midline	Infectious for 6 days from onset of rash Post-herpetic neuralgia is a common complication in the elderly
Mastitis	Inflammation and infection of the breast tissue Risk factors: Breastfeeding, cracked/sore nipple, nipple piercing	Painful breast swelling	Fever Unilateral breast oedema Erythema and tenderness Breast feels hard on palpation Ipsilateral axillary LN ± Purulent nipple discharge	A firm red tender lump indicates an abscess
Acute pericarditis	Causes: Idiopathic, infection (usually viral), post-MI, RA, SLE, hypothyroidism, Dressler's syndrome, malignancy, trauma	Sharp persistent central chest pain ± Radiation to left arm or abdomen Worse on inspiration, coughing and lying flat Relieved by sitting forward	Fever ± Pericardial friction rub	Shortness of breath and raised JVP suggests a pericardial effusion or cardiac tamponade
Pulmonary embolism	Commonly a venous thrombus Risk factors: Immobility, recent surgery, pregnancy, puerperium, malignancy, family history, COCP, HRT, thrombophilia, smoking, obesity	Pleuritic chest pain Breathlessness ± Haemoptysis ± Dizziness ± Syncope	Fever Tachycardia Tachypnoea Hypotension Raised JVP Pleural rub ± Swollen calf (suggests DVT)	Recurrent emboli may cause chronic breathlessness

Diagnosis	Background	Key symptoms	Key signs	Additional information
Pneumothorax	Common causes: Trauma, spontaneous, pre-existing lung disease, iatrogenic Risk factors: Smoking, subpleural bleb/bullae, tall thin stature Recurrence is common	Pleuritic chest pain Acute breathlessness	*On affected side:* Reduced chest expansion Reduced air entry Hyper-resonant to percussion	Small pneumothoraces may be asymptomatic A deviated trachea away from the affected side indicates a tension pneumothorax
Oesophageal achalasia (See Dysphagia)				
Prinzmetal angina **(Variant angina)**	Coronary artery spasm IHD may be present Risk factors: Smoking, insulin resistance	Circadian episodes of chest pain at rest Frequent in the morning Syncope	Signs often absent	Associated with ventricular arrhythmias and sudden death
Bornholm disease **(Devil's Grip)**	Myositis due to Coxsackie virus Affects chest wall and abdominal muscles Usually young adults Summer and autumn epidemics Faecal–oral route transmission Self-limiting within 2 wks	Malaise Severe episodic stabbing/cramping pain in the side of the chest Runny nose Sore throat Nausea/vomiting ± Abdominal pain	Fever Unilateral pain Intercostal tenderness on palpation	
Aortic dissection	Longitudinal tear in aortic wall Age 50–70 yrs Risk factors: Hypertension, aortic aneurysm, trauma, smoking, Marfan's/Ehler's Danlos syndrome, biscupid aortic valve	Acute severe sharp chest pain Radiates to back Pain migrates with progressive dissection ± Chest pain	Sweating Pallor BP difference >20 mmHg between each arm Aortic regurgitation (≈50%) Distal arterial occlusion (e.g. limb ischaemia, abdominal pain)	
Hypertrophic obstructive cardiomyopathy	Abnormal LVH and wall stiffness Results in LV outflow obstruction Autosomal dominant ≈50% cases are sporadic Often presents in young adulthood	Shortness of breath on exertion Palpitations Syncope	Jerky pulse Prominent A wave in JVP Late systolic thrill at lower-left sternal edge Pansystolic murmur at apex (MR)	Ventricular arrhythmias and sudden death are common
Acute myocarditis	Middle-age Commonest cause: Infection (e.g. Coxsackie virus)	Asymptomatic or mimics MI Central chest pain Fatigue Shortness of breath Palpitations	Fever Tachycardia Soft S1 and S4 gallop Heart failure	
Dressler's syndrome	Myocardial necrosis Formation of cardiac autoantibodies Occurs days/months post-MI or heart surgery	Recurrent fever Malaise Pleuritic chest pain Radiation to left shoulder Shortness of breath	Pericardial friction rub ± Pleural effusion	Refer urgently to cardiology Can be complicated by pericardial effusion or cardiac tamponade

Cough

Diagnosis	Background	Key symptoms	Key signs	Additional information
Bronchiolitis	Usually due to Respiratory Syncytial Virus Age <1 yr Common in winter Droplet spread Self-limiting	Coryzal symptoms Poor feeding Shortness of breath Cough	Hyperinflated chest Tachypnoea >50 breaths/min Tachycardia >160 bpm Hyper-resonant chest percussion Widespread fine crackles Wheeze	Dehydration or respiratory distress warrants an emergency admission
Acute bronchitis	Inflammation confined to bronchi Usually viral Common pathogens: Influenza, rhinoviruses, RSV, *Haemophilus influenzae* Risk factors: Smoking, dusty or damp environment Self-limiting within 3 wks	Persistent cough (± sputum) ± Pleuritic or retrosternal pain ± Headaches ± Myalgia	Normal respiratory examination or Wheeze ± Fever	Focal chest signs (e.g. crepitations) and systemic upset suggest pneumonia

Diagnosis	Background	Key symptoms	Key signs	Additional information
Chronic obstructive pulmonary disease (Chronic bronchitis or emphysema)	Progressive airways obstruction Little or no reversibility FEV1 <80% predicted FEV1/FVC <70% Age >40 yrs Causes: Smoking, occupational pollutants, alpha-1 anti-trypsin deficiency	Cough and sputum on most days Lasts ≥3 months over 2 successive years Breathless on exertion ± Weight loss	Tachypnoea Hyperinflated chest Reduced chest expansion Quiet breath sounds Wheeze Resonant on percussion ± Accessory muscle use ± Cyanosis ± Flapping tremor	
Asthma (See Acute breathlessness)				
Croup (Acute laryngotracheitis)	Usually a viral infection Affects larynx and trachea Commonly children 1–3 yrs age Autumn and spring epidemics Self-limiting	Cough Coryzal symptoms Noisy breathing Symptoms worse at night ± Shortness of breath	Barking cough Stridor Hoarse cry/voice ± Intercostal recession ± Tachypnoea	
Pneumonia	Common in winter months Risk factors: Age (infants and elderly), immunosupression, alcohol abuse, i.v. drug use, pre-existing lung disease, IHD, hospitalisation, aspiration	Vary depending on pathogen	*Common signs in all subtypes:* Haemoptysis Bronchial breathing Coarse crackles over affected lobe Focally reduced air entry Dull percussion over affected lobe Pleural rub	Lower lobe pneumonia is a common cause of upper abdominal pain
Common subtypes in the UK:				
Streptococcus pneumoniae (Pneumococcal)	Gram-positive diplococcus Often preceded by viral URTI Common in children, elderly, immunocompromised, COPD	Initially dry cough Pleuritic chest pain ± Rusty coloured sputum	Acute onset fever ± Herpes labialis	Pneumoccocal vaccine available for high-risk groups
Haemophilus influenzae	Common in children and pre-existing lung disease	Initially dry cough Pleuritic chest pain ± Yellow–green sputum	Acute onset fever	
Viral pneumonia in children	Common causes: Respiratory Syncytial Virus and adenoviruses Usually self-limiting	Gradual onset symptoms Coryzal symptoms	Low-grade fever <39°C Skin rash Wheeze	
Viral pneumonia in adults	Common cause: Influenza Type A Droplet spread Usually self-limiting	Headache Myalgia Dry cough ± Photophobia	Low-grade fever <39°C	Influenza vaccine available for high-risk groups
Mycoplasma pneumoniae	Atypical pneumonia Children and elderly Epidemic every 4 yrs	Coryzal symptoms Fatigue ± Dry cough or purulent sputum	Fever Wheeze Polyarthritis	Fatigue can persist for months post-infection
Chlamydia psittaci (Psittacosis)	Transmission via infected bird excrement (e.g. parrots, budgerigars) Incubation up to 2 wks	Diffuse headache Myalgia Dry cough Diarrhoea Vomiting	Fever ± Hepatosplenomegaly ± Abdominal macular rash	
Staphylococcus aureus	Widespread lung infection with bilateral cavitation Usually follows influenza Commonly children, elderly, i.v. drug users, immunocompromised	Acute onset Productive cough Blood/purulent sputum Pleuritic chest pain	Fever Chest expansion reduced	A high swinging fever suggests empyema
Legionnaire's disease	Aerobic gram-negative bacillus M:F ratio: ≈2:1 Highest incidence among travellers Air-borne in water droplets Thrives in water tanks <60°C (e.g. air-conditioning systems, bath spa's)	Coryzal symptoms Dry cough (may turn productive) Diarrhoea Vomiting Anorexia Haematuria	Fever Confusion Wheeze	

Diagnosis	Background	Key symptoms	Key signs	Additional information
Gastro-oesophageal reflux disease (See Chest pain)				
Chronic sinusitis (Chronic rhinosinusitis)	Paranasal sinus inflammation Nose frequently involved Common pathogens: Anaerobes, gram-negative bacteria, *Staphylococcus aureus* Common risk factors: URTI, smoking, asthma, allergy, DM, swimming, dental infection	≥1 of the following lasting >12 wks: Facial pain/pressure Purulent nasal discharge Post-nasal drip Reduction/loss of smell ± Cough ± Bad breath (halitosis) ± Malaise ± Headache ± Upper toothache	Tenderness over sinuses Facial pain worse on stooping Normal respiratory examination ± Fever	Consider ENT referral
Lung carcinoma (Bronchial carcinoma)	Incidence increases >40 yrs age Risk factors: Smoking, industrial pollutants (e.g. arsenic, iron oxide, asbestos, radiation)	Chronic cough Haemoptysis Chronic breathlessness Chest or shoulder pain Weight loss	Cachexia Anaemia Clubbing Supraclavicular or axillary LN Gynaecomastia ± Chest signs (e.g. consolidation, effusion) ± Metastases (e.g. bony tenderness, confusion, hepatomegaly)	Histological subtypes: Squamous ≈30% Adenocarcinoma ≈30% Small (oat cell) ≈25% Large cell ≈15% Alveolar cell <1%
Bronchiectasis	Chest infection leads to permanently dilated bronchi/ bronchioles Usual onset in adulthood Common causes: Post-infective, RA, bronchial obstruction, hypogammaglobulinaemia, congenital (e.g. cystic fibrosis)	Chronic daily cough Duration months to years Copious purulent sputum Haemoptysis Malaise Pleuritic chest pain	Fever Coarse inspiratory crackles Wheeze ± Clubbing (severe disease)	
Inhaled foreign body (See Stridor)				
Pulmonary tuberculosis	Chronic granulomatous disease Droplet spread			Notifiable disease Refer to respiratory specialist
Stage of infection:				
Primary TB	Initial infection produces a pulmonary lesion (Ghon focus) Ghon focus usually heals and calcifies Immunity develops	Usually asymptomatic or Non-specific (e.g. fatigue, weight loss)	Signs may be absent	Complications include widespread dissemination of TB (Miliary TB)
Post-primary TB	Reactivation of primary TB Ghon focus enlarges with lymphatic spread ± Extra-pulmonary organ spread (e.g. bone) Risk factors: Close contact with TB patient, children, vagrants, foreign travel, immunocompromise, malnutrition	Symptoms develop late: Productive cough Fatigue Weight loss Anorexia Night sweats ± Haemoptysis	Fever Cervical LN Variable respiratory signs ± Erythema nodosum	Respiratory signs vary (e.g. upper-lobe crackles, effusion) Complications include widespread dissemination of TB (Miliary TB)

Diagnosis	Background	Key symptoms	Key signs	Additional information
Cystic fibrosis	Autosomal recessive Common in Caucasians Associated with: Pancreatic insuffiency, DM, liver disease, male infertility Median survival >40 yrs age	*Neonatal symptoms:* Steatorrhoea Poor feeding *Child or adult symptoms:* Chronic cough Purulent sputum Weight loss Steatorrhoea ± Haemoptysis	*Neonatal signs:* Failure to pass meconium within 24 h of birth (meconium ileus) Prolonged jaundice Failure to thrive *Child or adult signs:* Recurrent LRTI Bilateral coarse crackles Wheeze Clubbing Nasal polyps Rectal prolapse	Morbidity and mortality are mainly associated with bronchiectasis and cor pulmonale
Measles	Acute viral infection Droplet spread Commonly children <6 yrs age Incubation up to 14 days Highly contagious Usually self-limiting	Coryzal symptoms Dry cough Red watery eyes Followed by onset florid rash	High-grade fever >39°C Conjunctivitis Discrete maculopapular rash Becomes blotchy and confluent Spreads from head/neck to trunk and limbs Rash lasts ≈3 days Koplik spots on buccal cheek mucosa (pathognomonic)	Notifiable disease Infectious up to 5 days after onset of rash Complications include: Bronchopneumonia, otitis media, encephalitis Higher risk if immunocompromised
Pertussis (Whooping cough)	Caused by *Bordetella pertussis* Highest incidence in infants Droplet spread Incubation up to 10 days	Coryzal symptoms last ≈2 wks Followed by >3 wks dry cough Cough associated with cyanosis, exhaustion and/or vomiting	Severe paroxysms of coughing Normal respiratory signs between coughing bouts ± Inspiratory whoops ± Subconjunctival haemorrhages	Notifiable disease Patients remain infectious for up to 5 days after starting antibiotics Cough may last ≥3 months post-infection
Pneumocystis carinii pneumonia	Opportunistic infection Associated with immunosupression AIDS-defining illness CD4 count often <200 cells/mm³	Dry cough Breathless on exertion Chest pain ± Sweats ± Weight loss	Fever Tachypnoea Normal breath sounds or Bilateral crackles and wheeze	Consider hospital admission
Listeriosis	Gram-positive bacillus Risk factors: Meat pâtés, soft cheese, unpasteurised milk, raw vegetables, sheep At-risk groups: Pregnancy, neonate, elderly, immunocompromised Healthy individuals can be asymptomatic	Headache Myalgia Cough Diarrhoea Vomiting Malaise Sore throat	Fever Conjunctivitis Bronchial breathing Coarse crackles over affected lobe Focally reduced air entry Dull percussion over affected lobe Pleural rub ± Vaginitis (in pregnancy)	Infection carries a high risk of miscarriage, preterm labour and/or stillbirth Listeriosis can cause meningo-encephalitis

Haemoptysis

Diagnosis	Background	Key symptoms	Key signs	Additional information
Pulmonary oedema (See Acute left ventricular failure)				
Pneumonia (See Cough)				
Lung carcinoma (Bronchial carcinoma)	Incidence increases >40 yrs age Risk factors: Smoking, industrial pollutants (e.g. arsenic, iron oxide, asbestos), radiation	Chronic cough Haemoptysis Chronic breathlessness Chest or shoulder pain Weight loss	Cachexia Anaemia Clubbing Supraclavicular or axillary LN Gynaecomastia ± Chest signs (e.g. consolidation, effusion) ± Metastases (e.g. bony tenderness, confusion, hepatomegaly)	Histological subtypes: Squamous ≈30% Adenocarcinoma ≈30% Small (oat cell) ≈25% Large cell ≈15% Alveolar cell <1%

Diagnosis	Background	Key symptoms	Key signs	Additional information
Pulmonary embolism	Commonly a venous thrombus Risk factors: Immobility, recent surgery, pregnancy, puerperium, malignancy, family history, COCP, HRT, thrombophilia, smoking, obesity	Pleuritic chest pain Breathlessness ± Haemoptysis ± Dizziness + Syncope	Fever Tachycardia Tachypnoea Hypotension Raised JVP Pleural rub ± Swollen calf (suggests DVT)	Recurrent emboli may cause chronic breathlessness
Bronchiectasis	Chest infection leads to permanently dilated bronchi/bronchioles Usual onset in adulthood Common causes: Post-infective, RA, bronchial obstruction, hypogammaglobulinaemia, congenital (e.g. cystic fibrosis)	Chronic daily cough Duration months to years Copious purulent sputum Haemoptysis Malaise Pleuritic chest pain	Fever Coarse inspiratory crackles Wheeze ± Clubbing (severe disease)	
Pulmonary tuberculosis (See Cough)				
Aspergilloma	Inhalation of fungal spores Causes fungal ball (mycetoma) growth within a lung cavity Spores present in soil and decaying vegetation Risk factor: Pre-existing lung cavitation (e.g. TB, sarcoidosis)	Usually asymptomatic or Cough Lethargy ± Weight loss	Normal respiratory examination	Haemoptysis can be torrential
Wegener's granulomatosis	Necrotizing granulomatous vasculitis Peak onset 35–55 yrs age Affects any organ Common organs: Ears, nose, throat, lungs, kidneys	Vary depending on organs involved *Common symptoms:* Malaise Runny nose Hearing loss Cough Shortness of breath	Vary depending on organs involved *Common signs:* Fever Conjunctivitis Epistaxis Nasal sores/ulcers Hoarse voice Haematuria Skin rash (e.g. blisters, nodules)	
Goodpasture's syndrome	Autoimmune vasculitis Results in: Anti-GBM antibodies, progressive glomerulonephritis and pulmonary haemorrhage Usually young Caucasian men	Shortness of breath Chest pain Nausea/vomiting Rigors Weight loss	Tachypnoea Cyanosis Bibasal inspiratory crackles	Respiratory and/or renal failure are the commonest causes of mortality Haemoptysis can be torrential

Palpitations

Diagnosis	Background	Key symptoms	Key signs	Additional information
Panic disorder	History of discrete episodes of anxiety (panic attacks) Intense subjective fear with symptomatic manifestations Unanticipated attacks Variable in frequency Attack lasts <1 h Chronic anxiety >1 month Anxiety related to subsequent attacks or effects of attack Agoraphobia may co-exist ≈50% develop depression	Fast palpitations Chest discomfort/pain Shortness of breath Dizziness Nausea/vomiting Numbness and tingling "Fear of losing control"	No physical signs between attacks *During an attack:* Hyperventilation Sweating Sinus tachycardia Hypertension Severe anxiety Affect congruent with mental state Fear of death/illness ± Suicidal ideation	Exclude alcohol/drug misuse

Diagnosis	Background	Key symptoms	Key signs	Additional information
Generalised anxiety disorder	Usually chronic persistent anxiety Excessive or unrealistic worry Inappropriate to the situation Affects daily functioning Associated with stress and depression	Fast palpitations Shortness of breath Dizziness Nausea/vomiting Numbness and tingling "Fear of losing control" Poor concentration Insomnia Urinary frequency Frequent or loose bowel motions Erectile dysfunction	Hyperventilation Sweating Sinus tachycardia Hypertension Severe anxiety Fear of death/illness Postural hand tremor	Exclude alcohol/drug misuse
Sinus tachycardia	Common causes: Emotion, exercise, infection, MI, heart failure, anaemia, hypovolaemia, pregnancy, thyrotoxicosis, caffeine, pain	Palpitations	Regular pulse rate Regular pulse volume Heart rate >100 bpm	
Atrial fibrillation	Prevalence increases >50 yrs age M>F Common causes: Idiopathic, hypertension, LVH, IHD, infection, mitral valve stenosis, excess alcohol, thyrotoxicosis, cardiomyopathy	Asymptomatic in ≈20% Intermittent or persistent palpitations ± Dizziness ± Chest pain ± Breathlessness	Irregularly irregular pulse rate Irregular pulse volume Cardiac apex rate > pulse rate	Absent P wave on ECG
Extrasystoles (Ectopic beats)	Isolated beats due to early depolarisation Focus origin outside of SA node (e.g. atrial muscle, ventricle) Usually benign Heart disease often absent Precipitated by excess alcohol or caffeine	Asymptomatic or "Heart misses a beat" intermittently	Irregularly irregular pulse rate Irregular pulse volume Signs usually disappear on moderate exercise	Frequent ventricular ectopics can induce VF (R on T phenomenon) Consider a cardiology referral if frequent ectopics or history of heart disease Ventricular ectopics are common post-MI
Supraventricular tachycardia	Abnormal focus above the ventricles Usual onset child or early adulthood Atria contract >150 bpm	Fast palpitations Start and stop abruptly Duration minutes to hours ± Dizziness + Chest pain ± Breathlessness	Fast and regular pulse rate >140 bpm	Sustained symptomatic SVT requires urgent admission Normal QRS complex on ECG
Menopause (See Amenorrhoea/ Oligomenorrhoea)				
Hyperthyroidism (Thyrotoxicosis)	Primary or secondary Age 20–50 yrs M:F ratio: ≈1:9 Causes: Graves' disease, thyroiditis, toxic nodule, amiodarone Eye changes suggest Graves' disease (e.g. exophthalmos)	Fast palpitations Hyperactivity Sweating Weight loss despite increased appetite Diarrhoea Heat intolerance ± Oligo/amenorrhoea	Tachycardia Lid lag Hair thinning or alopecia Fine postural hand tremor Warm peripheries Gynaecomastia Neck lump Neck lump moves up on swallowing Brisk reflexes ± AF ± Dull percussion over sternum ± Psychosis	*Consider thyrotoxic crisis if:* Fever Delirium Coma Seizures Jaundice Vomiting

Stridor

Diagnosis	Background	Key symptoms	Key signs	Additional information
Croup (Acute laryngotracheitis)	Usually a viral infection Affects larynx and trachea Commonly children aged 1–3 yrs Autumn and spring epidemics Self-limiting	Cough Coryzal symptoms Noisy breathing Symptoms worse at night ± Shortness of breath	Barking cough Stridor Hoarse cry/voice ± Intercostal recession ± Tachypnoea	
Inhaled foreign body	Foreign body can lodge at any level Right bronchus commonly affected	Vary depending on size of foreign body *Common symptoms:* Acute onset stridor Acute onset cough/spluttering	Stridor	Small foreign bodies can present late with chronic cough and chest infection
Laryngomalacia	Congenitally flaccid larynx collapses during respiration Onset a few weeks post-birth Symptoms typically become worse in the first year Usually resolves by 18–24 months Associated with reflux disease	Noisy breathing Worse on lying supine, feeding and crying	High-pitched stridor	
Laryngeal carcinoma	Commonly squamous cell Age >50 yrs M>F Risk factors: Smoking and alcohol	Persistent hoarseness Chronic cough ± Dysphagia ± Sore throat	Cervical LN Stridor (late sign)	Hoarseness >4 wks requires ENT referral to exclude malignancy
Acute epiglottitis	Swollen epiglottis Commonest cause: *Haemophilus influenza* type B (Hib) Children aged 1–8 yrs or adults	Acute onset symptoms over hours Severe sore throat Painful swallow (odynophagia) Unable to swallow fluids Malaise	Toxic appearance Drooling Upright forward posture High-grade fever >39°C Cervical LN Stridor (late sign)	DO NOT examine throat due to risk of complete airway obstruction
Diphtheria	Infection caused by *Corynebacterium diphtheriae* toxin Pseudomembrane formation Droplet spread or skin contact Prevalent in developing countries	Purulent/bloody nasal discharge Dysphagia ± Skin blisters and ulcers	Neck oedema ("Bull neck") Neck LN *Cutaneous signs:* Ruptured blisters on legs, feet/hands "Punched out" ulcers covered by a dark pseudomembrane and haemorrhagic base	Notifiable disease Complications include: Muscle paralysis, cardiac arrhythmia, airway obstruction

Chapter 5
Abdomen

Upper abdominal mass

Diagnosis	Background	Key symptoms	Key signs	Additional information
Hepatomegaly	Causes: Metastases, venous congestion, haematological, infection, metabolic, cysts, autoimmune	Vary and depend on underlying cause Common symptoms: Lethargy Anorexia RUQ pain or discomfort	Palpable RUQ mass Extends towards LIF Smooth or irregular on palpation ± Tenderness on palpation	Tongue-like extension of the right lobe (Riedel's lobe) is a normal variant Normal liver span: ≈10 cm in women ≈12 cm in men
Splenomegaly	Causes: Portal hypertension, haematological, infection, cysts, metastases Associated with hypersplenism	Vary and depend on underlying cause *Common symptoms:* Lethargy Bleeding (e.g.epistaxis)	Palpable LUQ mass Extends towards RIF Unable to palpate above the mass Notched leading edge Moves on inspiration Dull to percussion	A palpable spleen is at least double the normal size
Abdominal aortic aneurysm (AAA)	Weakness of the infra-renal aortic wall Causes irreversible vessel dilatation Age 40–70 yrs M>F Risk factors include: Family history, smoking, hypertension, increasing age, PVD Aneursyms >5 cm diameter are high risk	Often asymptomatic or Vague abdominal or back pain Upper abdominal pulsation	Expansile pulsatile mass above umbilicus ± Bruit ± Weak/absent peripheral pulses	Severe lumbar pain may indicate a leaking or dissecting aneurysm
Gastric Carcinoma (See Upper Abdominal Pain)				
Intussusception	Invagination of bowel segment into adjacent distal segment Usually affects ileo-caecal segment Causes bowel obstruction Commonly 3 months to 2 yrs age Often idiopathic	Acute onset Severe colicky abdominal pain Intermittent every 10–15 min May appear well between attacks Inconsolable screaming epsiodes Vomiting	Sausage-shaped abdominal mass "Redcurrant jelly" stools	Emergency paediatric referral
Pyloric stenosis	Diffuse hypertrophy and hyperplasia of the pylorus and antrum Commonly infants 2–8 wks old M>F Persistent vomiting causes hypokalaemia and hypochloraemic alkalosis	Recurrent projectile vomiting Vomitus contains undigested food Persistent hunger Weight loss Infrequent or absent bowel movement	Dehydration Lethargy Visible stomach peristalsis Palpable "olive" mass in RUQ or epigastrum	Symptoms in adults are rare and gastric carcinoma should be excluded

Differential Diagnosis in Primary Care, 1st edition. By Nairah Rasul and Mehmood Syed. Published 2009 by Blackwell Publishing, ISBN: 978-1-4051-8036-8

Diagnosis	Background	Key symptoms	Key signs	Additional information
Polycystic kidneys	Autosomal dominant Bilateral renal cyst formation Can lead to chronic renal failure Most present in adulthood Cysts can also occur in the liver, spleen, pancreas Associated with Berry aneurysms	Acute onset loin pain Haematuria	Hypertension Tender mass in both flanks	
Volvulus	Twisted loop of bowel Causes acute or intermittent bowel and vessel obstruction Commonly infants and elderly Risk factors: Constipation and gut malrotation	Acute colicky abdominal pain Constipation Vomiting	Tachycardia Abdominal distension ± Tender abdominal mass	An acute abdomen (i.e. peritonitis) suggests ischaemic bowel and perforation
Abdominal hernia (See Lower abdominal mass)				

Lower abdominal mass

Diagnosis	Background	Key symptoms	Key signs	Additional information
Pregnancy	History: Postive pregnancy test, missed period, missed pill, unprotected sex	Amenorrhoea Gradual lower abdominal swelling Breast tenderness Urinary frequency Fatigue ± Nausea/vomiting ± Constipation ± Galactorrhoea	*Palpable uterus:* Suprapubic at 12–14 wks Umbilical ≈20 wks	
Constipation	Common in children and elderly Causes include: Low fibre diet, dehydration, immobility, drugs, pregnancy, anal pain, intestinal obstruction, IBS, hypothyroidism, neuromuscular	≤2 bowel motions a week or Firm hard stools difficult to pass Lower abdominal pain/discomfort Abdominal bloating ± Nausea ± "Overflow" diarrhoea ± Urinary retention	Mild abdominal distension Palpable faecal loading in LIF ± Loaded rectum on PR	Explore any emotional or behavioural issues in children
Abdominal hernia				A tender irreducible hernia requires urgent surgical review
Subtypes:				
Para-umbilical hernia	M<F Risk factors: Weak abdominal muscles, multiparity, obesity	Intermittent abdominal mass Appears on standing or straining	Mass above or below umbilicus Palpable cough impulse	High risk of incarceration or strangulation
Incisional hernia	Occurs months/years post-surgery Risk factors: Wound infection or haematoma, obesity, chronic cough/straining	Progressive abdominal mass Appears on standing or straining	Often large Lies over an abdominal scar Palpable cough impulse	
Umbilical hernia	Commonly premature infants Benign Usually resolves by 5 yrs age if <1 cm diameter	Umbilical mass worse on crying	Easily reducible Palpable cough impulse	
Epigastric hernia	Midline swelling defect in the linea alba, above the umbilicus Commonly young men	Intermittent epigastric mass Appears on standing or straining ± Epigastric pain	Abdominal swelling above umbilicus Often small Palpable cough impulse	High risk of incarceration or strangulation
Spigelian hernia	Swelling lateral to the rectus sheath	Discomfort/ache on exertion	Palpable cough impulse	

Diagnosis	Background	Key symptoms	Key signs	Additional information
Urinary retention	Bladder outlet obstruction or detrusor muscle dysfunction			
Subtypes:				
Acute urinary retention	Commonly in elderly M>F Causes: Prostatic obstruction, constipation, drugs, UTI, pain, urethral stricture, bladder carcinoma, clot retention, spinal cord compression, alcohol	Sudden inabilty to pass urine Severe lower abdominal pain	Suprapubic tenderness Firm tender suprapubic mass Dull to percussion Normal perineal sensation	Absent or impaired perineal sensation indicates cauda equina compression
Chronic urinary retention	Incomplete bladder emptying Causes: BPH, pelvic malignancy, neurological, urethral obstruction	Insidious onset No abdominal pain Nocturnal enuresis Overflow urinary incontinence	Firm non-tender suprapubic mass Dull to percussion Normal perineal sensation	
Uterine fibroid **(Uterine leiomyoma)**	Benign tumour of the myometrium Affects ≈1 in 4 women Usually grow slowly under oestrogen stimulation Vary in size and number Risk factors: Afro-Carribean, perimenopause, family history, nulliparity Regress at menopause unless on HRT	Up to 50% are asymptomatic or Heavy prolonged periods Intermenstrual bleeding Pressure symptoms (e.g. urinary frequency) ± Subfertility	*PV examination:* Enlarged irregular uterus ± Firm pelvic mass	Complications include pelvic pain due to fibroid torsion or degeneration Malignancy is rare
Colorectal carcinoma (See Rectal bleeding)				
Ascites	Due to portal hypertension and liver failure Causes: Liver cirrhosis, malignancy, heart failure, pancreatitis Risk factors: Alcohol abuse, hepatitis B/C, autoimmune, genetic (e.g. Wilson's disease), drugs	Swollen abdomen Poor appetite Shortness of breath	Abdominal distension Shifting dullness ± Jaundice ± Muscle wasting	Complications include spontaneous bacterial peritonitis
Ovarian carcinoma	Approximately 90% are epithelial Most cases are sporadic Commonly postmenopausal women Risk factors: Obesity, early menarche, late menopause, nulliparity, breast cancer COCP is protective	Gradual abdominal swelling Bloating Lower abdominal/pelvic pain Early satiety Urinary frequency	Palpable abdominal or pelvic mass ± Ascites	Often presents with late symptoms <1% ovarian tumours are androgen-secreting (arrhenoblastoma) and associated with hirsutism
Pelvic abscess	Acute or chronic inflammation Abscess lies anterior to the rectum Risk factors: Colitis, appendicitis, diverticulitis, PID, post-abortion	Malaise Nausea Lower abdominal pain Diarrhoea ± Urinary frequency	Fever Deep tenderness in lower abdomen Localised tenderness on PV or PR exam ± Bulging of anterior rectal wall	

Upper abdominal pain

Diagnosis	Background	Key symptoms	Key signs	Additional information
Non-ulcer dyspepsia **(Functional dyspepsia)**	Commonest type of dyspepsia No underlying organic pathology Associated with IBS	Heartburn Bloating Belching Early satiety Nausea	Normal abdominal examination	
Gastroenteritis (See Diarrhoea)				
Duodenal ulcer **(Peptic ulcer disease)**	Commonest peptic ulcer Usually benign M>F Middle-age Risk factors: *H. pylori*, drugs (e.g. NSAID), family history, smoking	Epigastric pain before meals Relieved by eating, or drinking milk Worse at night Weight gain	Mild epigastric tenderness ± Haematemesis ± Melaena	Acute severe generalised abdominal pain suggests a perforation
Gastric ulcer **(Peptic ulcer disease)**	Often involves the lesser curve Benign or malignant Commonly elderly M>F Risk factors: *H. pylori*, NSAID, stress, smoking, delayed gastric emptying	Epigastric pain after meals Worse in the day Relieved by vomiting Weight loss	Mild epigastric tenderness ± Haematemesis ± Melaena	
Gall stone obstruction	Common sites: CBD, gallbladder neck, cystic duct, Ampulla of Vater M<F Risk factors for gall stones: Caucasian, obesity, middle-age, multiparity, ileal resection, haemolysis, liver disease Stones often pass spontaneously	Often asymptomatic or History of fatty food intolerance History of indigestion Acute onset RUQ or epigastric pain Severe recurrent pain Radiates to right shoulder blade or back Duration minutes to hours Resolves abruptly Nausea/vomiting Normal bowel habit	No fever ± RUQ tenderness ± Jaundice	Complications include: Cholecystitis, pancreatitis, obstructive jaundice
Acute cholecystitis	Gallbladder inflammation Often due to biliary stone impaction M<F Risk factors for gall stones: Caucasian, obesity, middle-age, multiparity, ileal resection, haemolysis, liver disease	Malaise Acute onset severe RUQ or eigastric pain Radiates to right shoulder tip Constant pain Worse on inspiration Vomiting Normal bowel habit	Fever Tachycardia Shallow respirations Local guarding over RUQ Positive Murphy's sign ± Jaundice ± RUQ mass	
Lower-lobe pneumonia (See Cough)				
Diabetic ketoacidosis **(DKA)**	Hyperglycaemia and ketoacidosis Often due to Type I DM Develops over hours/days Commonly young adults Risk factors: Infection, inadequate insulin, non-comliance, undiagnosed DM, illness (e.g. MI, CVA), alcohol abuse, medication (e.g. steroids, beta blockers)	Acute onset symptoms Fatigue Malaise Weight loss Shortness of breath Polyuria and frequency Polydipsia Nausea/vomiting Non-specific abdominal pain	Severe dehydration Tachypnoea Tachycardia Ketotic breath ± Confusion ± Infection (e.g. URTI, UTI) *Abnormal urinalysis:* Glycosuria ± Ketonuria	
Ulcerative colitis (See Diarrhoea)				
Crohn's disease (See Diarrhoea)				

Diagnosis	Background	Key symptoms	Key signs	Additional information
Intestinal obstruction	Obstruction can be functional (ileus) or mechanical Causes: Post-surgery, hernia, adhesions, stricture (e.g. Crohn's), malignancy, faecal impaction, inflammation	Vary depending on level of obstruction *High-level obstruction:* Abdominal pain after eating Early vomiting Late constipation Passing flatus *Low-level obstruction:* Late vomiting Early constipation Not passing flatus	Vary depending on type and level of obstruction *High-level obstruction:* Minimal abdominal distension Early dehydration *Low-level obstruction:* Gross abdominal distension Late dehydration *Functional obstruction:* Absent or "tinkling" bowel sounds *Mechanical obstruction:* Loud hyperactive bowel sounds	Guarding and abdominal tenderness indicate peritonitis
Hepatitis (See Jaundice)				
Myocardial infarction (See Chest pain)				
Polycystic kidneys	Autosomal dominant Bilateral renal cyst formation Can lead to chronic renal failure Most present in adulthood Cysts can also occur in the liver, spleen, pancreas Associated with Berry aneurysms	Acute onset loin pain Haematuria	Hypertension Tender mass in both flanks	
Sickle cell crisis	Red blood cell sickling causes small vessel occlusion or haemolysis Due to sickle cell disease (HbSS) High-risk groups: West African, African-Carribean, Asian, Mediterranean, Middle-eastern Triggers: Infection, cold, hypoxia, dehydration, physical stress	Acute onset pain Severity of pain is variable May mimic an acute abdomen	Site of pain depends on organs involved *Common signs:* Mild fever Bony pain Swollen hands/feet Priapism	
Acute pancreatitis	Autodigestion of the pancreas releases pancreatic enzymes into the peritoneum Common causes: Gall stones, alcohol abuse, idiopathic Other causes: Trauma, mumps, autoimmune, hyperlipidaemia, drugs (e.g.steroids)	Acute onset severe epigastric pain Radiates through to back Constant pain Relieved by sitting forward Nausea/vomiting	Hypovolaemic shock: Hypotension Tachycardia Dehydration Shallow breathing Abdominal guarding or tenderness Absent bowel sounds ± Jaundice ± Grey Turner's sign (flank bruising) ± Cullen's sign (peri-umbilical bruising)	
Gastric carcinoma	Age >55 yrs M:F ratio: ≈3:1 Risk factors: Smoking, *H. pylori* infection, family history, atrophic gastritis, pernicious anaemia, blood group A High prevalence in Japan and China	New onset dyspepsia >4 wks Weight loss Vomiting Anorexia Abdominal pain	Anaemia Epigastric mass Melaena Palpable left supraclavicular LN (Virchow's node)	

Diagnosis	Background	Key symptoms	Key signs	Additional information
Henoch-Schönlein purpura	Commonest allergic vasculitis IgA-mediated Small vessel vasculitis Affects: Kidneys, abdomen, skin Commonly 3–10 yrs age M:F ratio: ≈2:1 Often follows recent URTI Usually self-limiting within several weeks	Skin rash Lower limb arthralgia Colicky abdominal pain Vomiting Diarrhoea (can be bloody) Haematuria	Mild fever Symmetrical purpuric rash ± Slightly raised Non-itchy Affects buttocks and back of legs Swollen tender lower-limb joints *Abnormal urinalysis:* Haematuria Proteinuria	Renal complications are more frequent and severe in older children
Abdominal hernia (See Lower abdominal mass)				
Intussusception	Invagination of bowel segment into adjacent distal segment Usually affects ileo-caecal segment Causes bowel obstruction Commonly 3 months to 2 yrs age Often idiopathic	Acute onset symptoms Severe colicky abdominal pain Intermittent every 10–15 min May appear well between attacks Inconsolable screaming epsiodes Vomiting	Sausage-shaped abdominal mass "Redcurrant jelly" stools	Emergency paediatric referral
Bowel ischaemia/infarction	Middle-aged or elderly Causes: Mesenteric arterial embolism or thrombosis, hernia strangulation, adhesions, volvulus, intussusception Risk factors: Recent MI, AF, aortic valve disease/prosthesis, hernia Associated with IHD and PVD	Acute onset abdominal pain Colicky in nature Bright red rectal bleeding ± History of abdominal pain after meals	Tachycardia Hypotension Abdominal distension Abdominal guarding Absent bowel sounds	Admit for immediate surgical assessment
Acute cholangitis	Bile duct infection due to bile stasis Common pathogens: Gram-negatives, (e.g. *E. coli*, *Klebsiella*) Risk factors: Gall stone obstruction, thick bile, CBD stricture, malignancy, ERCP, parasites (e.g. liver fluke)	Malaise Nausea Rigors Abdominal pain	*Charcot's triad* of signs: Jaundice High swinging fever Tender RUQ ± Septic shock ± Confusion	Emergency admission for i.v. antibiotics
Hypercalcaemia	Common causes: Primary hyperparathyroidism, malignancy, CRF Risk of cardiac arrhythmia due to shortened QT interval	Vary depending on severity *Common symptoms:* Lethargy Low mood Polyuria Polydipsia Constipation Muscle weakness	Confusion Dehydration	Long-term complications include renal stones and chondrocalcinosis Avoid thiazides
Chronic pancreatitis	Irreversible pancreatic fibrosis Results in malabsorption and DM Causes include: Alcohol (≈60%), pancreatic duct obstruction, cystic fibrosis, haemachromatosis, hypercalcaemia, drugs, trauma	Chronic or intermittent epigastric pain Often severe Radiates through to back Relieved by sitting forward Steatorrhoea Anorexia Weight loss Nausea/vomiting	Mild or moderate epigastric tenderness	Pain is a common complication Beware opiate addiction
Carcinoma of the pancreas (See Jaundice)				
Addison's disease	Primary adrenal insufficiency Commonest cause: Autoimmune Precipitated by: Trauma, stress, infection, infarction Autoimmune diseases often co-exist (e.g. IDDM, Graves' disease)	Insidious onset symptoms Lethargy Weakness Anorexia Weight loss Nausea/vomiting Diarrhoea ± Severe abdominal pain	Vitiligo Postural hypotension *Hyperpigmentation of:* Palmar creases Buccal mucosa Axillae Scars	Abrupt withdrawal or reduction in chronic steroids can provoke an Addisonian crisis Shock and hypoglycaemia warrant an emergency admission

Diagnosis	Background	Key symptoms	Key signs	Additional information
Acute intermittent porphyria	Mostly dominant inheritance Enzyme deficiency in haem synthesis Toxic accumulation of haem precursors Onset post-puberty Attacks precipitated by drugs: Alcohol, anaesthetics, antibiotics, COCP, anticonvulsants	Intermittent attacks Anxiety Colicky abdominal pain Vomiting Constipation	Fever Hypertension Psychosis Seizures Hypotonia Peripheral neuropathy Urine turns deep red on standing	Cutaneous porphyria causes skin blistering on sun exposure

Lower abdominal pain

Diagnosis	Background	Key symptoms	Key signs	Additional information
Cystitis	M<F Often due to *E. coli* in all ages Risk factors include: Renal stones, enlarged prostate, sexual intercourse, pregnancy, DM, GU instrumentation, structural anomalies, menopause	Suprapubic discomfort Urine frequency or Incontinence or retention (elderly) Dysuria Cloudy and offensive urine Nausea/vomiting	Fever Suprapubic tenderness ± Confusion (in elderly) *Abnormal urinalysis:* Nitrites Leucocytes ± Haematuria	Consider referral in males and young children May progress to pyelonephritis
Dysmenorrhoea (See Women's health)				
Mittelschmerz	Physiological pain Related to ovulation Spontaneously resolves	Dull iliac fossa pain Onset around mid-cycle Relieved by analgesia	Normal PV examination Normal abdominal examination	
Constipation	Common in children and elderly Causes include: Low-fibre diet, dehydration, immobility, drugs, pregnancy, anal pain, intestinal obstruction, IBS, hypothyroidism, neuromuscular	≤2 bowel motions a week or Firm hard stools difficult to pass Lower abdominal pain/discomfort Abdominal bloating ± Nausea ± "Overflow" diarrhoea ± Urinary retention	Mild abdominal distension Palpable faecal loading in LIF ± Loaded rectum on PR	Explore any emotional or behavioural issues in children
Acute urinary retention	Commonly elderly M>F Causes: Prostatic obstruction, constipation, drugs, UTI, pain, urethral stricture, bladder carcinoma, clot retention, spinal cord compression, alcohol	Sudden inabilty to pass urine Severe lower abdominal pain	Suprapubic tenderness Firm tender suprapubic mass Dull to percussion Normal perineal sensation	Absent or impaired perineal sensation indicates cauda equina compression
Mesenteric adenitis	Non-specific inflammation of the mesenteric LN Commonly children Follows a recent viral URTI	Poorly localised abdominal pain Headache ± Diarrhoea	High-grade fever >39°C Generalised LN Moderate tenderness in RIF No rebound tenderness Normal PR exam	
Acute pyelonephritis	Kidney infection Infection from bladder or blood Usually *E. coli* M<F Risk factors include: Renal stones, enlarged prostate, pregnancy, sex, DM, GU instrumentation, structural anomalies	Onset pain over 1–2 days Unilateral or bilateral loin pain Rigors Malaise Anorexia Vomiting Urinary frequency Dysuria Cloudy offensive urine ± Suprapubic pain	Fever Unilateral or bilateral loin tenderness Suprapubic tenderness ± Frank haematuria ± Leucocytes/nitrites	Complications include perinephric abscess and septicaemia Admit if obstruction suspected
Gilmore's groin	Tear of adductor thigh muscles Close to attachment to pubic bone May follow acute injury or gradual muscle overuse Typically sportsmen (e.g. footballers)	Progressive groin pain Worse on running, twisting, turning, coughing Sore or stiff groin post-exertion	Groin pain on adducting hips No hernia	

Diagnosis	Background	Key symptoms	Key signs	Additional information
Appendicitis	Appendix often retrocaecal Commonly 10–20 yrs age Key symptoms often absent in the very young and old	Central colicky abdominal pain Migrates to RIF after hours/days Worse on movement and coughing Becomes progressively worse Anorexia Vomiting	Low-grade fever <39°C Tachycardia Rebound tenderness or guarding in RIF (McBurney's point) Palpation of LIF induces RIF pain (Rovsing's sign) ± Anterior tenderness on PR examination ± Trace haematuria	Consider ectopic pregnancy
Ureteric obstruction	Commonest cause is calculi Peak onset age 30–50 yrs M:F ratio: ≈3:1 Risk factors for calculi: Anatomical anomalies, hypercalcaemia, hyperoxaluria, hyperuricaemia, dehydration, UTI ≈80% calculi pass spontaneously May take up to 3 wks Recurrence is common	Acute onset severe loin pain Colicky in nature Radiates to ipsilateral groin and tip of penis or labia (renal colic) Nausea/vomiting Haematuria (can be frank) ± Hesitancy	Unilateral pain Restless due to pain Sweating Normal abdominal examination ± Mild loin tenderness *Abnormal urinalysis:* Haematuria	Renal calculi with fever or rigors indicates superimposed infection and is a urological emergency
Pelvic inflammatory disease	Acute or chronic infection Often polymicrobial Risk factors: STIs, IUCD, uterine instrumentation, post-termination, miscarriage Associated with: Subfertility, ectopic pregnancy, chronic pelvic pain	May be asymptomatic or Bilateral lower abdominal pain Deep dyspareunia Vaginal discharge Menorrhagia Dysmenorrhoea	Lower abdominal tenderness ± Fever *Pelvic examination:* Bilateral adnexal tenderness Cervical excitation *Speculum examination:* Mucopurulent cervical discharge Cervicitis	Pregnant women should be urgently referred to gynaecology
Ectopic pregnancy	Occurs in the first trimester Commonest site: Fallopian tube History of positive pregnancy test Common risk factors: PID, IUCD, progesterone-only pill, previous pelvic surgery, advancing age	Acute or chronic onset symptoms Unilateral constant iliac fossa pain Followed by dark vaginal bleeding Usually scanty in volume ± History of missed period	Tachycardia Hypotension (in extremis) Lower abdominal rebound tenderness *PV examination:* Cervical excitation Cervical os closed	Emergency gynaecology admission
Diverticulitis	Acute inflammation of one or more diverticulae Usually affects sigmoid colon Age >50 yrs ≈75% people with diverticulosis remain asymptomatic	Typically LIF pain Intermittent or constant pain Constipation (few have diarrhoea) Anorexia Nausea/vomiting ± PR bleed	Fever Tachycardia Tenderness in LIF Tenderness on PR examination ± Palpable LIF tender mass	Consider admission for i.v. antibiotics Approximately one third of patients develop complications: Perforation, fistulae, abscess, obstruction
Ovarian cyst torsion	Torsion of the pedicle compromises blood supply Possbile history of intermittent pelvic pain	Acute onset symptoms Severe unilateral iliac fossa pain Nausea/vomiting	Fever Tachycardia Abdominal tenderness Guarding Tenderness on PV examination	Ovarian cysts may haemorrhage or rupture and present similarly
Red degeneration of fibroid (See Abdominal pain in pregnancy)				

Constipation

Diagnosis	Background	Key symptoms	Key signs	Additional information
Diet and lifestyle	Common in the elderly and children Usually chronic Dietary factors: Poor fluid and soluble-fibre intake Lifestyle factors: Inactivity, ignoring urge to defaecate	Lower abdominal pain/discomfort Abdominal bloating ± Nausea ± "Overflow" diarrhoea	Mild abdominal distension Palpable faecal loading in the LIF ± Loaded rectum on PR	Consider painful perianal conditions

Diagnosis	Background	Key symptoms	Key signs	Additional information
Pregnancy (See Lower abdominal mass)				
Medication	Common drugs: Opiate analgesics, iron, aluminium-containing antacids, anticholinergics, ACE inhibitors	Onset constipation after taking medication	Mild abdominal distension Palpable faecal loading in the LIF ± Loaded rectum on PR	
Irritable bowel syndrome	No underlying structural pathology Symptoms present >6 months Age 20–40 yrs M<F Precipitated by: Stress, menses, antibiotics, gastroenteritis Food intolerance is common	Continuous or intermittent symptoms Altered bowel motion Constipation and/or diarrhoea Colicky central or LIF pain Relieved by defaecation Associated with a "morning rush" Bloating Rectal mucus discharge No rectal bleeding ± Tenesmus	Apyrexial ± Non-specific mild abdominal tenderness	
Diverticular disease	Commonly >50 yrs age Prevalence increases with age Common with Western diet Affects any part of the colon Usually sigmoid colon	Left-sided lower abdominal pain Colicky in nature Relieved by defaecation or flatus ± Worse on eating Bloating Flatulence Alternate constipation and diarrhoea ± Painless rectal bleeding (can be profuse)	Apyrexial ± Mild tenderness in the LIF	Fever and tachycardia suggest diverticulitis Asian patients have predominantly right-sided diverticulae and may present with RIF pain
Emotional/behavioural problems	Toddlers acquiring toilet skills and school-age children Painful defaecation leads to witholding and further constipation History of: Parental anxiety Coercive toilet training Family conflict	≤2 bowel motions a week or Firm hard stools difficult to pass ± Pain on defaecation ± Faecal soiling ± Encoperesis	Palpable faecal loading in the LIF Large faecal mass in the rectum No anal stenosis or fissure Normal sacrum	
Acquired hypothyroidism	Age >60 yrs M<F Causes: Autoimmune, thyroiditis, TSH deficiency, postpartum, thyroidectomy, neck radiation, iodine deficiency, drugs (e.g. amiodarone, carbizamole) Associated with: High cholesterol/triglycerides and anaemia	Lethargy Weight gain Low mood Cold intolerance Menorrhagia	Deep hoarse voice Slow cognition (e.g. poor memory) Dry coarse skin Thinning of hair Bradycardia Slow-relaxing tendon reflexes ± Goitre	Beware myxoedema in the elderly: Puffy eyes, hands and feet Cerebellar ataxia Hypothermia Seizures ± Coma
Colorectal carcinoma (See Rectal bleeding)				
Intestinal obstruction	Obstruction can be functional (ileus) or mechanical Causes: Post-surgery, hernia, adhesions, stricture (e.g. Crohn's), malignancy, faecal impaction, inflammation	Vary depending on level of obstruction *High-level obstruction:* Abdominal pain after eating Early vomiting Late constipation Passing flatus *Low-level obstruction:* Late vomiting Early constipation Not passing flatus	Vary depending on type and level of obstruction *High-level obstruction:* Minimal abdominal distension Early dehydration *Low-level obstruction:* Gross abdominal distension Late Dehydration *Functional obstruction:* Absent or "tinkling" bowel sounds *Mechanical obstruction:* Loud hyperactive bowel sounds	Guarding and abdominal tenderness indicate peritonitis

Diagnosis	Background	Key symptoms	Key signs	Additional information
Hypercalcaemia	Common causes: Primary hyperparathyroidism, malignancy, CRF Risk of cardiac arrhythmia due to shortened QT Interval	Vary depending on severity *Common symptoms:* Lethargy Low mood Polyuria Polydipsia Constipation Muscle weakness	Dehydration Confusion	Long-term complications include: Renal stones and chondrocalcinosis Avoid thiazides
Hirschsprung's disease	Congenital Aganglionic segment of rectum May extend to the colon Commonly neonates Occasionally presents in childhood M:F ratio: ≈4:1 Associated with Down's syndrome	Delayed passage of meconium >48 h post-birth Chronic constipation Abdominal discomfort Early satiety	Failure to thrive Distended abdomen Empty rectum	Paediatric referral

Diarrhoea

Diagnosis	Background	Key symptoms	Key signs	Additional information
Gastroenteritis	Viral or faecal–oral transmission Common risk factors: Poor hygiene, undercooked food, contaminated food or water	Frequent passing of loose stools Abdominal cramps Relieved by defaecation ± Nausea/vomiting	Often normal abdominal examination ± Dehydration	Dysentery and all cases of food poisoning are notifiable Beware dehydration and renal failure Advise contraceptive pill users to use additional precautions
Common subtypes in UK:				
Norovirus	Common cause of "winter vomiting" Affects hospitals, schools, nursing homes, cruise ships Risk factors: Contaminated water, shellfish Incubation 24–60 h Usually self-limiting within 1–2 days Immunity is short-lived	Watery diarrhoea Vomiting Intermittent abdominal cramps	Fever	
Rotavirus	Children <5 yrs age and elderly Winter and spring epidemics Risk factor: Poor hygiene Incubation 2–3 days Self-limiting	Watery diarrhoea Vomiting Coryzal symptoms Lactose intolerance	Low-grade fever <39°C	Transient lactose intolerance can last for weeks
Clostridium difficile	Common gut commensal Risk factors: Hospitalisation, antibiotic use within the past 2 months Incubation 1–7 days	Watery yellow diarrhoea Intermittent abdominal cramps	Fever	Complications include: Pseudomembranous colitis and toxic megacolon
Campylobacter	Often *C. jejuni* and *C. coli* Commonly children and young adults Risk factors: Unpasteurised milk, infected water, raw poultry Incubation 2–5 days Self-limiting	Watery and bloody diarrhoea Nausea Malaise Severe intermittent abdominal cramps	Persistent fever Non-specific abdominal tenderness	Associated with post-infectious IBS
Salmonella	Often *Salmonella enteritidis* Commonly elderly and infants Risk factors: Infected meat (e.g. poultry, beef), water, eggs, vegetables Incubation 6–72 h Usually self-limiting within 4–7 days	Intermittent abdominal cramps Vomiting ± Blood in stool	Fever No rash ± Generalised abdominal tenderness	Associated with post-infectious IBS

Diagnosis	Background	Key symptoms	Key signs	Additional information
Cryptosporidium	Protozoan parasite Commonly children and HIV patients Risk factors: Contaminated livestock, personal contact (e.g. nurseries, patients, contaminated food/water) Incubation 4–12 days Usually self-limiting in the immunocompetent	Green offensive diarrhoea Malaise Intermittent abdominal cramps ± Blood in stool	Low-grade fever <39°C	Persistent cryptosporidia-positive stool >1 month is AIDS-defining
Escherichia coli	Strain O157 Common in travellers Risk factors: Undercooked beef, unpasteurised milk, raw vegetables Incubation 12–72 h Usually self-limiting within 2 wks	Diarrhoea ± Blood in stool 2–3 days later Nausea/vomiting Intermittent abdominal cramps	Apyrexial or low-grade fever <39°C	Haemolytic uraemic syndrome occus in ≈7% of children: Pallor Weight gain/oedema Oliguria
Shigella (Bacillary dysentery)	>90% due to *Shigella sonnei* Typically affects children Risk factors: Contaminated fruit, vegetables, shellfish Incubation 1–3 days Usually self-limiting within 3–7 days	Acute onset watery diarrhoea Followed by bloody diarrhoea Intermittent abdominal cramps Tenesmus Malaise	Fever Lower abdominal tenderness Normal or increased bowels sounds	Notifiable disease
Drugs	Common causes: Alcohol, laxatives, antibiotics, antacids, cimetidine, thiazides, digoxin	Onset diarrhoea after taking medication	Apyrexial Normal abdominal examination	
Toddler's diarrhoea	Associated with rapid bowel transit Benign Children between ages 1–5 yrs Usually resolves by age 6 yrs Excerbated by excess fruit juices/squash	Persistent loose stools after meals Between 3–10 motions a day Stool consistency varies Undigested food in the stool	Well child Normal abdominal examination Normal weight gain	
Overflow constipation (See Constipation)				
Irritable bowel syndrome	No underlying structural pathology Symptoms present >6 months Age 20–40 yrs M<F Precipitated by: Stress, menses, antibiotics, gastroenteritis Food intolerance is common	Continuous or intermittent symptoms Altered bowel motion Constipation and/or diarrhoea Colicky central or LIF pain Relieved by defaecation Associated with a "morning rush" Bloating Rectal mucus discharge No rectal bleeding ± Tenesmus	Apyrexial ± Non-specific mild abdominal tenderness	
Diverticular disease	Commonly >50 yrs age Prevalence increases with age Common with Western diet Affects any part of the colon Usually sigmoid colon	Left-sided lower abdominal pain Colicky in nature Relieved by defaecation or flatus ± Worse on eating Bloating Flatulence Alternate constipation and diarrhoea ± Painless rectal bleeding (can be profuse)	Apyrexial ± Mild tenderness in the LIF	Fever and tachycardia suggest diverticulitis Asian patients have predominantly right-sided diverticulae and may present with RIF pain

Diagnosis	Background	Key symptoms	Key signs	Additional information
Coeliac disease (Gluten-sensitive enteropathy)	Gluten intolerance Villous atrophy and malabsorption Peak onset ages 9 months to 5 yrs and 40–60 yrs M<F Gluten stimulates IgA endomysial and transglutaminase antibodies Gluten foods: Barley, rye, wheat Requires a lifelong gluten-free diet Associated with: Osteoporosis, hyposplenism, IgA deficiency, Type I DM	At least one third are asymptomatic Symptoms occur after ingesting gluten Steatorrhoea Bloating Abdominal pain Abdominal distension Fatigue Anorexia Weight loss or failure to thrive	Anaemia Angular stomatitis Aphthous mouth ulcers ± Dermatitis herpetiformis	The risk of GI malignancy and GI T-cell lymphoma is reduced by a gluten-free diet
Lactose intolerance	Autosomal recessive Usually late onset in child or adulthood Level of lactose intolerance varies Transient intolerance also common Causes: Intestinal infection or inflammation	Acute onset watery diarrhoea Occurs hours after ingesting milk product Abdominal pain Bloating Flatulence Weight loss Symptoms improve on milk reduction or avoidance	Normal abdominal examination	
Traveller's diarrhoea				
Common subtypes:				
Giardiasis	Chronic diarrhoeal infection Causes carbohydrate and fat malabsorption Faecal–oral transmission Risk factors: Infected water, swimming, poor sanitation, daycare centres Prevalent in the tropics Incubation 1–2 wks Stool may be positive for cysts	Chronic or recurrent symptoms Loose watery offensive stools ± Explosive nature No blood or pus Upper/central abdominal cramps Bloating Offensive flatulence Anorexia Weight loss Malaise	Apyrexial Normal abdominal examination	
Typhoid and paratyphoid fever (Enteric fevers)	Caused by *Salmonella* strains *S. typhi* and *S. paratyphi* Faecal–oral transmission Risk factors: Contaminated food or water Incubation 3 days to 3 wks Prevalent in South America and Asia Multi-organ spread via the blood ≈1% become chronic carriers	*1st week:* Malaise Dry cough Anorexia Constipation *2nd week:* Diarrhoea Vomiting Abdominal pain ≥3 *wks:* Offensive green diarrhoea	Persistent high-grade fever >39°C Bradycardia *2nd week:* Abdominal distension Mild abdominal tenderness Rose spots (red macules) on the trunk Hepatomegaly ≥3 *wks:* Confusion	Notifiable disease Late complications include: Bowel haemorrhage and perforation
Amoebic dysentery	Parasitic infection of the colon Can spread to other organs ~90% are asymptomatic carriers Faecal–oral transmission Risk factors: Infected food/water Incubation days to years Symptoms often start years later Prevalence: South and Central America, West Africa, SE Asia	Slow onset intermittent diarrhoea Becomes profuse Blood and pus in stool Lower abdominal pain Anorexia	Fever Generalised abdominal or RIF tenderness ± RIF mass (amoeboma)	Complications include Amoeboma, severe colitis and liver abscess
Cholera	Bacterial infection Caused by *Vibrio cholerae* Risk factor: Contaminated water Incubation few hours to 5 days High prevalence: India, Bangladesh, Africa, Peru	Profuse watery diarrhoea Up to 1 litre per hour Vomiting	Fever Tachycardia Hypotension Rapid dehydration Sunken eyes	Notifiable disease Rapid dehydration is a leading cause of death

Diagnosis	Background	Key symptoms	Key signs	Additional information
Colorectal carcinoma	Age >45 yrs Prevalence increases with age Common risk factors: Family history, IBD, colorectal polyps, obesity, smoking Often metastasizes to the liver	Change in bowel habit for ≥6 wks Persistent frequent stools/ diarrhoea Bright red rectal bleeding or Dark blood mixed with stool Rectal mucus discharge Tenesmus Weight loss	Anaemia ± Palpable rectal mass ± Palpable iliac fossa mass	Refer for urgent colonoscopy
Crohn's disease (Inflammatory bowel disease)	Chronic disorder Relapsing and remitting disease Affects any part of the gut Usually terminal ileum and proximal colon Peak onset ages 15–30 yrs and 60–80 yrs Risk factor: Smoking Normal bowel between affected areas (skip lesions)	Chronic diarrhoea >2 wks Upper abdominal cramping pains Weight loss ± Rectal bleeding	Abdominal tenderness Aphthous oral ulcers RIF mass Perinanal disease (e.g.fistulae, skin tag, abscess) Anal stricture on PR examination ± Clubbing ± Erythema nodosum ± Pyoderma gangrenosum ± Red eyes (e.g. uveitis) ± Large joint arthritis	Admit if severe disease: Fever Tachycardia Severe abdominal tenderness or distension Motions >6 times/day Large rectal bleed
Ulcerative colitis (Inflammatory bowel disease)	Chronic disorder Relapsing and remitting disease Only affects rectum and/or colon Peak onset age 15–40 yrs Smoking is protective ≈4% have extra-intestinal disease Associated with: PSC and colorectal carcinoma	Gradual onset bloody diarrhoea Upper abdominal cramping pains ± Rectal mucus discharge ± Tenesmus (in proctitis)	Abdomen non-tender in mild disease ± Clubbing ± Erythema nodosum ± Pyoderma gangrenosum ± Red eyes (e.g. uveitis) ± Large joint arthritis	Admit if severe disease: Fever Tachycardia Severe abdominal tenderness or distension Motions >6 times/day Large rectal bleed Complications include: Toxic megacolon and haemorrhage
Hyperthyroidism (Thyrotoxicosis)	Primary or secondary Age 20–50 yrs M:F ratio: ≈1:9 Causes: Graves' disease, thyroiditis, toxic nodule, amiodarone Eye changes suggest Graves' disease (e.g. exophthalmos)	Fast palpitations Hyperactivity Sweating Weight loss despite increase appetite Heat intolerance ± Oligo/amenorrhoea	Tachycardia Lid lag Hair thinning or alopecia Fine postural hand tremor Warm peripheries Gynaecomastia Neck lump Neck lump moves up on swallowing Brisk reflexes ± AF ± Dull percussion over sternum ± Psychosis	Consider thyrotoxic crisis if: Fever Delirium Coma Seizures Jaundice Vomiting
Cystic fibrosis (See Cough)				
Chronic pancreatitis (See Upper abdominal pain)				
Carcinoid syndrome	5-HT (serotonin)–secreting tumour Usually of the appendix and small intestine Most are benign and asymptomatic A few metastasize to the liver This results in carcinoid syndrome Often presents late	Explosive watery diarrhoea Abdominal pain Wheeze (bronchospasm) Transient skin flushing Worse after alcohol and caffeine	*Right-sided heart failure due to:* Pulmonary stenosis Tricuspid regurgitation	

Diagnosis	Background	Key symptoms	Key signs	Additional information
Zollinger Ellison syndrome	Gastrin-secreting adenoma Usually of the pancreas Typically presents 20–60 yrs age Often sporadic History of persistent peptic ulcer >50% are malignant Multiple adenomas may be present ≈30% associated with MEN type I	Diarrhoea Steatorrhoea Epigastric pain Indigestion	Epigastric tenderness ± Anaemia ± Hepatomegaly (metastases) ± Melaena	
Whipple's disease	Chronic gut malabsorption Caused by *Tropheryma whippelii* Elderly males >50 yrs age Commonly Caucasian Multisystem disease Affects CNS, heart, eyes	Intermittent arthralgia Anorexia Weight loss Steatorrhoea Abdominal pain Flatulence Chronic cough Pleuritic chest pain	Intermittent low-grade fever <39°C Skin hyperpigmentation ± Generalised LN ± Anaemia	Polyarthralgia is transient and migratory

Groin swelling

Diagnosis	Background	Key symptoms	Key signs	Additional information
Inguinal hernia	M:F ratio: ≈8:1 Risk factors: Male gender, obesity, chronic cough, heavy lifting, constipation, prematurity in infants Onset acute or gradual			An irreducible hernia is at risk of vascular compromise and infarction (strangulation) If a hernia is very tender, seek an immediate surgical opinion
Subtypes:				
Indirect hernia	Commonly young adults or children Commonest inguinal hernia Enters via deep inguinal ring Exits via superficial inguinal ring May enter the scrotum or labia major	Progressive groin or scrotal swelling Usually unilateral Appears on standing or straining ± Localised pain ± "Dragging sensation" in scrotum	*On standing:* Visible groin or scrotal swelling Above and medial to pubic tubercle Palpable cough impulse Mobile swelling Unable to palpate above mass *On lying down:* ± Reducible Controlled by pressure over deep inguinal ring (above femoral pulse)	Exclude symptoms of bowel obstruction
Direct hernia	Commonly elderly Protudes through the posterior wall of the inguinal canal Rarely enters the scrotum	Progressive groin swelling Usually unilateral Appears on standing or straining ± Localised pain	*On standing:* Visible groin swelling Above and lateral to pubic tubercle Palpable cough impulse Mobile swelling Unable to palpate above mass *On lying down:* ± Reducible NOT controlled by pressure over deep inguinal ring	Exclude symptoms of bowel obstruction
Femoral hernia	M:F ratio: ≈1:4 Often middle-aged or elderly Enters via the femoral canal	Progressive groin swelling Usually unilateral Appears on standing or straining ± Localised pain	*On standing:* Visible groin swelling Below and lateral to pubic tubercle Mobile swelling Unable to palpate above mass ± Palpable cough impulse *On lying down:* ± Reducible Controlled by pressure over the femoral canal	Consider referral for hernia repair High risk of strangulation

Diagnosis	Background	Key symptoms	Key signs	Additional information
Inguinal lymphadenopathy	Local or general LN Causes: Infection and neoplasm Normal LN may be palpable in thin people Inguinal LN drain the leg, foot, perineum, lower trunk	*Common symptoms of infection:* Fever Malaise *Common symptoms of neoplasm:* Weight loss Lethargy	*Infectious LN:* Local or generalised Small numerous swellings Often tender Soft and mobile Not reducible *Neoplastic LN:* Local or generalised Non-tender swellings Large and rubbery or hard Not reducible ± Fixed to the skin ± Hepatosplenomegaly	Exclude genital tract infection
Sebaceous cyst (Epidermoid cyst)	Proliferation of epidermal cells in the dermis Benign Slow growth Commonly young adults M>F Common sites: Face, trunk, neck, extremities, scalp Often resolves spontaneously Often recur if not excised	Painless lump(s)	Skin-coloured Single or multiple Often round or oval Variable in size Firm subcutaneous nodule Central punctum Fixed to skin Not reducible Not pulsatile ± Uninfected foul cheese-like discharge	A tender and erythematous cyst suggests infection
Saphena varix	Incompetent valve at the sapheno–femoral junction Associated with varicosities of the long and short saphenous vein	Lump in the groin ± Leg discomfort after prolonged standing	*On standing:* Bluish groin swelling ("blow out") Usually unilateral Variable size Soft and compressible Palpable cough impulse Palpable fluid thrill on coughing ± Venous eczema and pigmentation of leg *Positive Trendelenburg test:* Swelling reducible on supine leg raise Controlled by groin pressure while standing Swelling reappears after removing pressure	
Undescended testicle (Cryptochordism)	Commonly male infants Age <1 yr Causes: Maldescent, ectopic, retraction Often unilateral Spontaneous descent usually complete by birth or before age 1 yr	Asymptomatic	*Ectopic/maldescended testis:* Immobile testis Lies outside scrotum (e.g. upper thigh, anterior abdominal wall, penile root, perineum) Underdeveloped scrotum *Retractile testis:* Mobile testis Lies at the neck of the scrotum Can be actively returned to scrotum Normal scrotum	Complications of ectopic and maldescended testes include: Infertilty, testicular trauma/torsion, testicular malignancy post-puberty Refer all cases of undescended testes >1 yr age
Lipoma	Adipose tumour Usually benign Slow growth Commonly adults Often multiple (lipomatosis) Common sites: Neck, trunk, upper arms, shoulders Does not occur on palms or soles Can occur in deeeper tissues	Painless lump(s)	Skin-coloured Single or multiple Often irregular in shape Usually <5 cm diameter Soft subcutaneous nodule Smooth normal skin surface Mobile Not reducible Not pulsatile	If >5 cm and rapid growth, refer to exclude liposarcoma

Diagnosis	Background	Key symptoms	Key signs	Additional information
Local skin abscess (See Pustules/Vesicles)				
Femoral artery aneurysm	May present with a distal thrombosis Can be associated with AAA	Usually asymptomatic	Expansile pulsatile groin swelling Lies midpoint below inguinal ligament	

Jaundice

Diagnosis	Background	Key symptoms	Key signs	Additional information
Physiological jaundice	Immature conjugation Increased erythrocyte breakdown Affects ≈50% of neonates Resolves within 10 days Risk factors: Prematurity and inadequate breastfeeding Can be toxic in preterm neonates	Poor feeding Sleepy	Onset jaundice day 2/3 post-birth	Persistently high unconguated bilirubin can cause kernicterus Jaundice within 24 h of birth or >10 days duration requires further investigation
Hepatitis	Viral infection			All types are notifiable Carriers of HBV and HCV are at risk of devoping cirrhosis and hepatocellular carcinoma
Subtypes:				
Hepatitis A	Children and young adults Faecal–oral transmission Incubation ≈2–6 wks Risk factors: Contaminated food/water High prevalence: Eastern Europe, Asia, Africa, Middle-East Chronic liver disease does not occur Lifelong immunity with IgG Self-limiting within 2 months	Asymptomatic or *Prodromal phase lasts 3–10 days:* Nausea Malaise Vomiting Anorexia RUQ discomfort/ache Diarrhoea *Followed by icteric phase lasts 1–3 wks:* Jaundice Dark urine Steatorrhoea	*Prodromal phase:* Low-grade fever <39°C Normal abdominal examination *Icteric phase:* Apyrexial Tender hepatomegaly ± Splenomegaly	Fulminant hepatitis is rare Occasionally jaundice persists for 12 wks
Hepatitis B	Transmission: Parenteral, sexual, vertical Long incubation 1–6 months At-risk groups: IVDU, homosexuals, healthcare workers High prevalence: Far East, Africa, Southern Europe ≈90% recover fully ≈10% become HBsAg carriers <1% develop fulminant hepatitis	*Acute infection:* Asymptomatic or As for Hepatitis A plus Skin rash Arthralgia *Chronic infection (carrier):* Asymptomatic or Malaise	*Acute infection:* Normal examination or Tender hepatomegaly ± Splenomegaly *Chronic infection (carrier):* Normal examination or Signs of cirrhosis	Symptoms can be more severe and prolonged than Hepatitis A
Hepatitis C	Transmission: Parenteral, sexual, vertical Incubation: 1–5 months Main risk group: IVDU High prevalence: South and East Asia, Eastern Europe, Japan Up to 85% become HCV carriers ≈30% carriers develop chronic liver disease after 15–20 yrs <1% develop fulminant hepatitis	>80% asymptomatic or Icteric phase as for Hepatitis A	Normal examination or Signs of cirrhosis	Initially LFTs may be normal despite progressive liver disease

Diagnosis	Background	Key symptoms	Key signs	Additional information
Hepatic carcinoma	Primary or secondary (metastases) Primary tumour is rare Commonly hepatocellular carcinoma Causes of HCC: Cirrhosis, chronic hepatitis B/C, drugs, parasites (e.g. schistosomiasis), toxins Metastases indicate late disease Common primary tumours metastasizing to liver: Lung, breast, GI	Anorexia Weight loss Malaise Upper abdominal pain	Irregular or nodular hepatomegaly Palpable left supraclavicular LN (Virchow's node) ± Ascites ± Jaundice ± *Metastatic symptoms:* Confusion Shortness of breath Bony pain	
Cirrhosis	Irreversible liver fibrosis and nodule formation M>F Common causes: Alcohol abuse, chronic hepatitis B/C, PBC, Wilson's disease, haemachromatosis, cryptogenic	Symptoms often few or vague Anorexia Gradual weight loss Fatigue	Bruising Clubbing Palmar erythema Dupuytren's contracture Spider naevi above waist Gynaecomastia Dilated peri-umbilical veins Hepatomegaly ± Splenomegaly *Late signs:* Jaundice Ascites Leukonychia Flapping tremor (encephalopathy) Small firm irregular or nodular liver	Complications: Oesophageal varices, ascites, encepalopathy, HCC, heptorenal syndrome Abnormal coagulation is a sensitive test of liver function
Gallstone obstruction (See Upper abdominal pain)				
Intrinsic haemolytic anaemia	Hereditary Common causes: Sickle cell disease, G6PD deficiency, spherocytosis, thalassaemia Life span of red blood cells <120 days Reticulocytosis >2% of RBCs	Vary depending on underlying cause	Mild or intermittent jaundice Anaemia Splenomegaly	
Malaria	Usually *Plasmodium falciparum* The most severe *Plasmodium* strain Causes haemolytic anaemia Incubation 7–14 days Usually presents within 2 months Endemic areas: SE Asia, Far East, sub-Saharan Africa Risk factors: Recent travel, airport staff	Recurrent fever Malaise Headache Anorexia Myalgia *Followed by:* Rigors Night sweats	Fever Anaemia Hepatosplenomegaly	Notifiable disease Warrants emergency admission Complications include: Cerebral malaria, hypoglycaemia, severe anaemia, pulmonary oedema, acute renal failure A single negative blood film does not exclude malaria
Carcinoma of head of the pancreas	≈60% of all pancreatic tumours Mostly ductal adenocarcinoma Age >60 yrs M>F Presents late Metastasizes early Risk factors: Alcohol, smoking, chronic pancreatitis, DM May present with: DVT, thrombophlebitis migrans, new onset DM, acute pancreatitis	Insidious onset Anorexia Weight loss Fatigue Pruritis Nausea/vomiting	Painless jaundice Palpable gallbladder Epigastric mass Palpable left supraclavicular LN (Virchow's node) Irregular hepatomegaly (metastases) ± Ascites	Courvoisier's Law: Painless jaundice and a palpable gallbladder is unlikely to be due to gallstones Refer urgently to upper GI surgeons

Diagnosis	Background	Key symptoms	Key signs	Additional information
Drug-induced jaundice	Common drugs: Rifampicin, paracetamol, isoniazid, chlorpromazine, methyl dopa, COCP Results in drug induced haemolysis or cholestasis	Onset jaundice after taking medication	Jaundice	
Right ventricular failure (See Chronic breathlessness)				
Acute cholangitis	Bile duct infection due to bile stasis Common pathogens: Gram-negatives, (e.g. *E. coli*, *Klebsiella*) Risk factors: Gall stone obstruction, thick bile, CBD stricture, malignancy, ERCP, parasites (e.g. liver fluke)	Malaise Nausea Rigors Abdominal pain	*Charcot's triad* of signs: Jaundice High swinging fever Tender RUQ ± Septic shock ± Confusion	Emergency admission for i.v. antibiotics
Primary biliary cirrhosis	Chronic progressive liver disease Affects intra-hepatic bile ducts Bile duct inflammation Results in cholestasis and cirrhosis Typical age at presentation ≈50 yrs M:F ratio: ≈1:9 AMA are 98% specific Associated with autoimmune disease	Pruritis RUQ pain/discomfort Fatigue	Hyperpigmentation Xanthomata Xanthelasma Hepatosplenomegaly *Late signs:* Jaundice Dark urine Steatorrhoea Cirrhosis	Recurrence can occur despite liver transplantation
Primary sclerosing cholangitis	Chronic progressive liver disease Affects intra and extra-hepatic bile ducts Bile duct fibrosis and stricture formation Results in cholestasis and cirrhosis Typical age at presentation 25–45 yrs M:F ratio: ≈2:1 AMA negative ≈80% ANCA positive Up to 75% have ulcerative colitis	Intermittent jaundice Pruritis RUQ pain/discomfort Fatigue Fever or night sweats Weight loss	Hepatomegaly ± Splenomegaly ± Hyperpigmentation ± Xanthomata *Late signs:* Jaundice Dark urine Steatorrhoea Cirrhosis	Recurrence can occur despite liver transplantation Complications include: Fat malabsorption, cholangiocarcinoma, bacterial cholangitis
Cholestatic jaundice of pregnancy	Intra-hepatic cholestasis Presents >20 wks gestation Associated with: Preterm delivery, fetal distress, perinatal mortality Resolves within 4 wks of delivery Recurs in up to 70% of pregnancies	Pruritis Steatorrhoea Anorexia Mild epigastric discomfort	Mild jaundice	Urgent referral to obstetrics COCP is permanently contraindicated Malabsorption of vitamin K can lead to bleeding or bruising
Leptospirosis (Weil's disease)	Caused by *Leptospira interrogans* From infected animal tissue or urine Commonly rats Transmission via direct contact through abraded skin or mucous membranes Incubation ≈7–14 days	Acute onset symptoms Severe headache Pain behind the eyes Lower-limb myalgia Nose bleeds Haemoptysis Nausea/vomiting Dry cough	Fever Photophobia Conjunctival haemorrhages Purpuric rash ± Tender hepatosplenomegaly	Complications include acute renal failure and GI haemorrhage

Diagnosis	Background	Key symptoms	Key signs	Additional information
Classical haemochromatosis	Autosomal recessive Excessive iron gut absorption M>F Women often present ≈10 yrs later than men Prevalent in Northern Europeans Affects pituitary, heart, liver, pancreas, joints	Chronic fatigue Arthralgia Erectile dysfunction	Slate-grey skin pigmentation Cirrhosis Heart failure (cardiomyopathy) New onset DM ± Testicular atrophy	First-degree relatives should be screened
Wilson's disease (Hepatolenticular degeneration)	Autosomal recessive Ceruloplasmin deficiency Results in toxic copper levels Affects CNS, liver, cornea, kidney Peak onset ages 10–13 yrs and young adults Initial presentation varies with age: Children usually present with liver disease and adults with neuropsychiatric signs	Dysphagia Personality change (e.g. disinhibition)	Cirrhosis Kayser-Fleischer rings (cornea) Blue nails Dysarthria Asymmetrical tremor Dyskinesis Delusions Dementia	First-degree relatives should be screened

Perianal pain

Diagnosis	Background	Key symptoms	Key signs	Additional information
Haemorrhoids	Submucous venous plexus swellings Prevalence increases with age Common risk factors: Constipation, pregnancy, family history, heavy lifting Usually painless unless thrombosed	Bright red rectal bleeding Blood separate from stool Blood occurs on wiping or Drips into pan after defeacation Rectal mucus Anal itch ± Perianal pain	Often painful PR examination	Complications include thrombosed or strangulated haemorrhoids
Subtypes:				
1st degree		As above	No visible or palpable anal swellings	
2nd degree		As above	Prolapsed bluish anal swellings Spontaneously reducible	
3rd degree		As above	Prolapsed bluish anal swellings Manually reducible	
4th degree		As above	Prolapsed bluish anal swellings Irreducible	
Anal fissure	Risk factors: Childbirth, constipation, Crohn's Usually self-limiting within 2 wks Internal sphincter spasm may delay healing	"Tearing" pain on defecation ± Minor bright red rectal bleeding on wiping	Very painful PR examination Visible anal mucosal tear Commonly in the midline posteriorly	
Pilonidal sinus	Sinus tract containing hair Usually occurs in the natal cleft Commonly young men <40 yrs age	Acute or chronic symptoms Often recurrent Painful and tender swelling ± Pus or bloody discharge	Sinus opening around natal cleft Pit in the midline of the sinus ± Tender on palpation ± Erythema (if infected)	A very tender fluctuant swelling indicates an abscess and warrants an urgent surgical referral
Perianal haematoma	Thrombosis of an anal vein Usually self-limiting over a few days	Acute onset symptoms Severe perianal pain ± Can be worse after straining	Tense bluish-black skin swelling Lies close to the anus Tender on palpation	

Diagnosis	Background	Key symptoms	Key signs	Additional information
Proctalgia fugax	Benign Occurs with intervals of weeks to months	Intermittent episodes Severe cramping pain of the rectum Lasts seconds to minutes No pain between attacks No rectal bleeding	Normal PR examination	
Coccydynia	M<F Risk factors: Childbirth, local trauma, bicycling, horse riding	Pain over coccyx Worse with constipation or sitting	Local tenderness over the coccyx	

Rectal bleeding

Diagnosis	Background	Key symptoms	Key signs	Additional information
Haemorrhoids	Submucous venous plexus swellings Prevalence increases with age Common risk factors: Constipation, pregnancy, family history, heavy lifting Usually painless unless thrombosed	Bright red rectal bleeding Blood separate from stool Blood occurs on wiping or Rectal mucus Anal itch ± Perianal pain	Often painful PR examination	Complications include thrombosed or strangulated haemorrhoids
Subtypes:				
1st degree		As above	No visible or palpable anal swellings	
2nd degree		As above	Prolapsed bluish anal swellings Spontaneously reducible	
3rd degree		As above	Prolapsed bluish anal swellings Manually reducible	
4th degree		As above	Prolapsed bluish anal swellings Irreducible	
Anal fissure	Risk factors: Childbirth, constipation, Crohn's Usually self-limiting within 2 wks Internal sphincter spasm may delay healing	"Tearing" pain on defecation ± Minor bright red rectal bleeding on wiping	Very painful PR examination Visible anal mucosal tear Commonly in the midline posteriorly	
Diverticular disease	Commonly >50 yrs age Prevalence increases with age Common with Western diet Affects any part of the colon Usually sigmoid colon	Left-sided lower abdominal pain Colicky in nature Relieved by defecation or flatus ± Worse on eating Bloating Flatulence Alternate constipation and diarrhoea ± Painless rectal bleeding (can be profuse)	Apyrexial ± Mild tenderness in the LIF	Fever and tachycardia suggests diverticulitis Asian patients have predominantly right-sided diverticulae and may present with RIF pain
Gastroenteritis (See Diarrhoea)				
Colorectal carcinoma	Age >45 yrs Prevalence increases with age Common risk factors: Family history, IBD, colorectal polyps, obesity, smoking Often metastasizes to the liver	Change in bowel habit for ≥6 wks Persistent frequent stools/diarrhoea Bright red rectal bleeding or Dark blood mixed with stool Rectal mucus discharge Tenesmus Weight loss	Anaemia ± Palpable rectal mass ± Palpable iliac fossa mass	Refer for urgent colonoscopy

Diagnosis	Background	Key symptoms	Key signs	Additional information
Ulcerative colitis (Inflammatory bowel disease)	Chronic disorder Relapsing and remitting disease Only affects rectum and/or colon Peak onset age 15–40 yrs Smoking is protective ≈4% have extra-intestinal disease Associated with: PSC and colorectal carcinoma	Gradual onset bloody diarrhoea Upper abdominal cramping pains ± Tenesmus (in proctitis) ± Rectal mucus discharge	Abdomen non-tender in mild disease ± Clubbing ± Erythema nodosum ± Pyoderma gangrenosum ± Red eyes (e.g. uveitis) ± Large-joint arthritis	Admit if severe disease: Fever Tachycardia Severe abdominal tenderness or distension Motions >6 times/day Large rectal bleed Complications include: Toxic megacolon and haemorrhage
Anticoagulant therapy	Common drugs: Warfarin, heparin, aspirin, clopidogrel Immunosupressants and cytotoxics can affect platelet count	History of anticoagulant use Bright red rectal bleeding or Melaena ± Haematuria	Normal abdominal examination	
Trauma	History of anal trauma	Rectal bleeding post recent trauma No change in bowel habit	Visible anal mucosal tear Non-tender abdomen	Consider non-accidental injury in children
Rectal prolapse	Partial or complete prolapse Commonly children and elderly Risk factors: Chronic constipation, straining, pregnancy, cystic fibrosis, malabsorptive disorder (e.g. coeliac)	Intermittent anal lump Occurs on defecation Lump may reduce on standing Rectal mucus discharge Faecal incontinence	Protruding anal mass Visible on sitting forward Concentric rings of rectal mucosa Rectal mucosa often engorged ± Reducible prolapse	
Intussusception	Invagination of bowel segment into adjacent distal segment Usually affects ileo–caecal segment Causes bowel obstruction Commonly 3 months to 2 yrs age Often idiopathic	Acute onset symptoms Severe colicky abdominal pain Intermittent every 10–15 min May appear well between attacks Inconsolable screaming epsiodes Vomiting	Sausage-shaped abdominal mass "Redcurrant jelly" stools	Emergency paediatric referral
Angiodysplasia	Occurs in any part of the gut Commonly affects right colon Typically elderly Associated with aortic stenosis	Intermittent episodes Painless bright red rectal bleeding Bleeding is mild or massive No change in bowel habit No weight loss	Anaemia Normal abdominal examination	
Bowel ischaemia/infarction	Middle-aged or elderly Causes: Mesenteric arterial embolism or thrombosis, hernia strangulation, adhesions, volvulus, intussusception Risk factors: Recent MI, AF, aortic valve disease/prosthesis, hernia Associated with IHD and PVD	Acute onset abdominal pain Colicky in nature Bright red rectal bleeding ± History of abdominal pain after meals	Tachycardia Hypotension Abdominal distension Abdominal guarding Absent bowel sounds	Admit for immediate surgical assessment

Chapter 6
Urinary Tract

Frequency

Diagnosis	Background	Key symptoms	Key signs	Additional information
Cystitis	M<F Often due to *E. coli* in all ages Risk factors include: Renal stones, enlarged prostate, sexual intercourse, pregnancy, DM, GU instrumentation, structural anomalies, menopause	Suprapubic discomfort Nausea/vomiting Urinary frequency or Incontinence or retention (elderly) Cloudy and offensive urine Dysuria	Fever Suprapubic tenderness ± Confusion (in elderly) *Abnormal urinalysis:* Nitrites Leucocytes ± Haematuria	Consider referral in males and young children May progress to pyelonephritis
Diabetes mellitus	Predisposing factors for DKA or HONK: Any infection, inadequate insulin or non-compliance, undiagnosed DM, illness (e.g. MI, CVA), drugs (e.g. beta-blockers, diuretics)			Inform DVLA Complications: CVA, MI, retinopathy, limb ischaemia, neuropathy, infections
Subtypes:				
Type I diabetes	Lack of endogenous insulin Commonly children or young adults Genetic predisposition Associated with autoimmune disease Risk of ketoacidosis Presentation is acute or subacute Longer history of symptoms	*Acute diabetic ketoacidosis:* Acute onset symptoms Fatigue Malaise Weight loss Polyuria and frequency Polydipsia Nausea/vomiting Non-specific abdominal pain *Subacute symptoms:* Fatigue Weight loss Polyuria and frequency Polydipsia Plus recurrent infections (e.g. boils, thrush, UTI)	*Acute diabetic ketoacidosis:* Severe dehydration Tachycardia Tachypnoea Ketotic breath ± Confusion ± Infection (e.g. URTI, UTI) *Abnormal urinalysis:* Glucose Ketones *Subacute signs:* *Abnormal urinalysis:* Glucose ± Ketones	DKA warrants emergency admission

Differential Diagnosis in Primary Care, 1st edition. By Nairah Rasul and Mehmood Syed. Published 2009 by Blackwell Publishing, ISBN: 978-1-4051-8036-8

Diagnosis	Background	Key symptoms	Key signs	Additional information
Type II diabetes	Reduced insulin secretion Increased insulin resistance Typical age >40 yrs Commonest type of diabetes Common risk factors: Obesity, South Asian, Afro-Carribean, male gender, family history, gestational DM, impaired glucose tolerance, metabolic syndrome, drugs (e.g. steroids) Not prone to ketoacidosis Presents insidiously or subacutely with HONK	*Insidious onset:* Weight loss Polyuria and frequency Polydipsia *Hyperosmolar non-ketotic coma:* Gradual onset symptoms over ≥1 wk Generalised weakness Lethargy ± Seizures	*Insidious onset:* Few signs may be present Glycosuria *Hyperosmolar non-ketotic coma:* Severe dehydration Tachycardia Confusion Drowsy Finger-prick glucose >30 mmol/litre ± Focal CNS signs (e.g. hemiparesis) ± Infection *Abnormal urinalyis:* Glucose No ketones	May eventually require insulin HONK warrants emergency admission High risk of DVT
Acute pyelonephritis	Kidney infection Infection from bladder or blood Usually *E. coli* M<F Risk factors include: Renal stones, enlarged prostate, pregnancy, sex, DM, GU instrumentation, structural anomalies	Onset pain over 1–2 days Unilateral or bilateral loin pain Rigors Malaise Anorexia Vomiting Urinary frequency Dysuria Cloudy offensive urine ± Suprapubic pain	Fever Unilateral or bilateral loin tenderness Suprapubic tenderness ± Frank haematuria ± Leucocytes/nitrites	Complications include perinephric abscess and septicaemia Admit if obstruction suspected
Benign prostatic hypertrophy	Glandular enlargement is testosterone-dependent Age >50 yrs >90% men aged ≥80 yrs have BPH Majority are asymptomatic Associated with detrusor muscle hypertophy and instability Outflow obstruction causes urge incontinence	*Bladder outlet obstruction:* Hesitancy Poor urine flow Terminal dribbling Incomplete bladder emptying Nocturia No dysuria ± *Bladder instability:* Frequency of small volumes Urgency	Enlarged prostate on PR examination Prostate firm and smooth Palpable median sulcus Normal anal sphincter tone Normal urinalysis ± Palpable bladder	A hard nodular prostate requires urgent investigation to exclude malignancy
Detrusor instability (Overactive bladder syndrome)	Common in elderly Risk factors: Multiple sclerosis, dementia, stroke, enlarged prostate	Urgency Urge incontinence Nocturia No dysuria No hesitancy	Normal abdominal examination Normal PV examination Normal urinalysis	
Pregnancy (See Lower abdominal mass)				
Generalised anxiety disorder (See Anxiety)				
Bladder stone	Middle-aged and elderly M>F Commonest cause is urinary stasis Risk factors: Bladder outlet obstruction, UTI, neurogenic bladder, urethral strcture, bladder diverticulum, foreign bodies	Suprapubic pain With sudden termination of micturition Followed by pain in tip of penis, scrotum and/or back Worse on movement Relieved by lying down Terminal frank haematuria Dysuria Hesitancy	*Abnormal urinalysis:* Haematuria ± Nitrites ± Leucocytes ± Palpable bladder	

Diagnosis	Background	Key symptoms	Key signs	Additional information
Prostatitis				All men should be referred post treatment to exclude a structural renal tract abnormality
Common subtypes:				PSA levels decrease wth treatment
Chronic bacterial prostatitis	Chronic or recurrent prostatitis for >3 months Men 40–70 yrs age Causes: Ascending urethral infection, intraprostatic urine reflux, lymphatic or haematogenous spread of infection Common pathogens: Gram-negative species (*E. coli, Klebsiella, Enterobacter*)	Chronic pelvic or perineal pain Ejaculatory pain Nocturia Urgency Dysuria Hesitancy Urethral discharge	Often apyrexial Normal abdominal examination Non-tender prostate on PR examination Enlarged prostate Testes non-tender on palpation	
Acute bacterial prostatitis	Men of all ages Causes: STI, UTI, lymphatic or haematogenous spread of infection, catheterisation Common pathogens: Gram-negative species, *Neiserria gonnorhoea, Chlamydia trachomatis*	Acute onset symptoms Pain in perineum or lower back Malaise Myalgia Arthralgia Nocturia Urgency Dysuria Hesitancy Incomplete voiding Urethral discharge	Fever Inguinal LN Lower abdominal tenderness Very tender prostate on PR examination Enlarged warm prostate Testes non-tender on palpation	If toxic or acute urinary retention admit for i.v. antibiotics
Urethral syndrome (Abacterial cystitis)	Commonly young women Caucasian Normal bladder Negative urine cultures Probable causes: Urethral stenosis or spasm, urethritis, stress, cold, nylon underwear, traumatic intercourse, allergy	Episodic or persistent symptoms Mild suprapubic discomfort Often relieved by voiding Urgency Daytime urinary frequency Minimal nocturia Dysuria ± Hesitancy	Normal urinalysis Normal PV examination	Exclude STI
Atrophic vaginitis	Post-menopausal women Falling oestrogen levels High vaginal pH Associated with recurrent UTI and vaginal infection	Vaginal/vulval soreness or itch Superficial dyspareunia Post-coital spotting Urgency Dysuria ± Urinary frequency ± Vaginal discharge	Normal abdominal examination Pale dry thin vaginal mucosa ± Contact bleeding ± Mucosal fissures	Significant post-menopausal bleeding warrants further investigation to exclude malignancy
Interstitial cystitis	Chronic relapsing/remitting condition Pancystitis results in bladder fibrosis and contraction Commonly middle-aged women ≈90% have large areas of bladder mucosal inflammation and damage (Hunner's ulcers)	Symptoms worse with menstruation Moderate suprapubic or pelvic pain Deep dyspareunia Nocturia Urgency Dysuria No hesitancy	Normal urinalysis	Consider specialist urology referral

Haematuria

Diagnosis	Background	Key symptoms	Key signs	Additional information
Cystitis (See Frequency)				
Bladder carcinoma	Commonest transitional cell carcinoma in the UK Age >65 yrs M:F ratio: ≈3:1 Risk factors: Smoking, urinary stasis, industrial exposure to aromatic amines (e.g. dye, rubber, paint, solvents), radiation Carcinoma in situ has a high rate of recurrence	Frank painless haematuria ± Urinary frequency ± Dysuria ± Urgency and incontinence	Often normal abdominal examination	Urgent referral to a urologist
Ureteric obstruction	Commonest cause is calculi Peak onset age 30–50 yrs M:F ratio: ≈3:1 *Risk factors for calculi:* Anatomical anomalies, hypercalcaemia, hyperoxaluria, hyperuricaemia, dehydration, UTI ≈80% calculi pass spontaneously May take up to 3 wks Recurrence is common	Acute onset severe loin pain Colicky in nature Radiates to ipsilateral groin and tip of penis or labia (renal colic) Nausea/vomiting Haematuria (can be frank) ± Hesitancy	Unilateral pain Restless due to pain Sweating Normal abdominal examination ± Mild loin tenderness *Abnormal urinalysis:* Haematuria	Renal calculi with fever or rigors indicates superimposed infection and is a urological emergency
Bladder stone	Middle-aged and elderly M>F Commonest cause is urinary stasis Risk factors: Bladder outlet obstruction, UTI, neurogenic bladder, urethral strcture, bladder diverticulum, foreign bodies	Suprapubic pain With sudden termination of micturition Followed by pain in tip of penis, scrotum and/or back Worse on movement Relieved by lying down Terminal frank haematuria Urinary frequency Dysuria Hesitancy	*Abnormal urinalysis:* Haematuria ± Nitrites ± Leucocytes ± Palpable bladder	
Prostate carcinoma	Commonly >65 yrs age Incidence increases with age Rare before 50 yrs age Risk factors: Family history, Afro-Carribean, high-fat diet, high androgen levels Metastasizes to seminal vesicles, bladder, bones, lung, liver, pelvic LN A normal PSA does not exclude carcinoma	Asymptomatic or Urinary frequency Urgency Hesitancy Poor urine stream No dysuria ± Urinary retention	Normal prostate on PR examination or Hard and nodular prostate	Urgent referral to a urologist
Polycystic kidneys	Autosomal dominant Bilateral renal cyst formation Can lead to chronic renal failure Most present in adulthood Cysts can also occur in the liver, spleen, pancreas Associated with Berry aneurysms	Acute onset loin pain	Hypertension Tender mass in both flanks	
Henöch-Schonlein purpura	Commonest allergic vasculitis IgA-mediated Small-vessel vasculitis Affects kidneys, abdomen, skin Commonly 3–10 yrs age M:F ratio: ≈2:1 Often follows recent URTI Usually self-limiting within several weeks	Skin rash Lower limb arthralgia Colicky abdominal pain Vomiting Diarrhoea (can be bloody) Haematuria	Mild fever Symmetrical purpuric rash ± Slightly raised Non-itchy Affects buttocks and back of legs Swollen tender lower-limb joints *Abnormal urinalysis:* Haematuria Proteinuria	Renal complications are more frequent and severe in older children

Diagnosis	Background	Key symptoms	Key signs	Additional information
Renal carcinoma	Pathology varies with age			
Common subtypes:				
Renal cell carcinoma	Usually malignant Age 60–80 yrs M:F ratlo: ≈2:1 Risk factors: Smoking, obesity, chronic dialysis, exposure to cadmium, asbestosis Cannon ball lung metastases are common	Recurrent fever Loin pain Painless haematuria (frank or microscopic) Anorexia Weight loss	Hypertension ± Palpable loin mass ± Left varicocele ± Bilateral leg oedema	Complications include polycythaemia and hypercalcaemia
Wilm's tumour (Nephroblastoma)	Malignant Sporadic or familial Commonly <5 yrs age Usually unilateral Cannon ball lung metastases are common	Vague abdominal pains Anorexia ± Haematuria	Fever Large abdominal mass ± Hypertension	
Anticoagulant therapy (See Rectal bleeding)				
Acute nephritic syndrome	Active glomerulonephritis Causes: Group A beta-haemolytic streptococci, post-viral, infective endocarditis, autoimmune (e.g. SLE), IgA nephropathy (Berger's), drug-induced, idiopathic	Oliguria Painless haematuria	Hypertension Facial oedema *Abnormal urinalysis:* Haematuria Proteinuria	Refer to a renal specialist Rapidly progressive glomerulonephritis can lead to end-stage renal failure within months
Blood dyscrasias	Causes include: Thrombocytopenia, haemophilia, sickle cell disease Often history of spontaneous bleeding	Vary depending on underlying cause *Symptoms may include:* Frank haematuria Severe loin pain in sickle cell disease	Vary depending on underlying cause *Signs may include:* Spontaneous bruising Loin tenderness Abdominal tenderness	
Trauma	History of blunt or penetrating trauma (e.g. RTA, fall, stabbing) Minor or major injury Pre-existing renal disease increases risk of renal injury	Vary depending on nature of injury *Symptoms may include:* Frank haematuria Loin pain	Vary depending on nature of injury *Signs may include:* Loin ecchymoses and/or abrasions Loin tenderness Tender ribs Abdominal tenderness	Consider admission for further assessment

Urinary incontinence

Diagnosis	Background	Key symptoms	Key signs	Additional information
Stress incontinence	Due to weak pelvic floor muscles M<F Prevalence increases with age Risk factors: Pregnancy, childbirth, post-menopause, pelvic prolapse, obesity	Frequent leakage of small amounts of urine Worse with coughing, laughing, sneezing, running No nocturia No dysuria No urgency	Normal abdominal examination ± Pelvic floor prolapse	
Cystitis (See Frequency)				
Detrusor instability (Overactive bladder syndrome)	Common in elderly Risk factors: Multiple sclerosis, dementia, stroke, enlarged prostate	Urgency Urge incontinence Nocturia No dysuria No hesitancy	Normal abdominal examination Normal PV examination Normal urinalysis	

Diagnosis	Background	Key symptoms	Key signs	Additional information
Benign prostatic hypertrophy (See Frequency)				
Bladder carcinoma (See Haematuria)				
Post-transurethral resection of prostate	Bladder sphincter damage History of recent TURP	Urgency Urge incontinence	Normal abdominal examination	
Impaired mobility	Common in elderly Unable to reach the toilet in time May be unaware of need to empty bladder	Urinary incontinence No dysuria	Normal abdominal examination Normal urinalysis	Exclude faecal impaction
Cauda equina syndrome	Common causes: Lumbar disc herniation, spinal tumour/ trauma, spinal abscess	Acute or gradual onset symptoms Low back pain Pain radiates to one or both legs Difficulty passing or stopping urine Faecal incontinence	Lower limb weakness Lower limb sensory deficit Absent lower limb reflexes Saddle anaesthesia ± Loss of anal tone and sensation	Emergency referral to neurosurgeons Delayed treatment can cause permanent neurological deficit

Urinary retention or oliguria

Diagnosis	Background	Key symptoms	Key signs	Additional information
Cystitis	M<F Often due to *E.coli* in all ages Risk factors include: Renal stones, enlarged prostate, sexual intercourse, pregnancy, DM, GU instrumentation, structural anomalies, menopause	Suprapubic discomfort Nausea/vomiting Urinary frequency or Incontinence or retention (elderly) Cloudy and offensive urine Dysuria	Fever Suprapubic tenderness ± Confusion (in elderly) *Abnormal urinalysis:* Nitrites Leucocytes ± Haematuria	Consider referral in males and young children May progress to pyelonephritis
Constipation (See Lower abdominal mass)				
Benign prostatic hypertrophy	Glandular enlargement is testosterone-dependent Age >50 yrs >90% men aged ≥80 yrs have BPH Majority are asymptomatic Associated with detrusor muscle hypertophy and instability Outflow obstruction causes urge incontinence	*Bladder outlet obstruction:* Hesitancy Poor urine flow Terminal dribbling Incomplete bladder emptying Nocturia No dysuria ± *Bladder instability:* Frequency of small volumes Urgency	Enlarged prostate on PR examination Prostate firm and smooth Palpable median sulcus Normal anal sphincter tone Normal urinalysis ± Palpable bladder	A hard nodular prostate requires urgent investigation to exclude malignancy
Urethral stricture	M>F Causes: GU instrumentation, catheterisation, urethral trauma, congenital, inflammation Associated with recurrent UTIs	Progressive reduction in urine flow Associated with straining Spraying or "double stream" of urine Terminal dribbling ± Urinary frequency ± Dysuria	Normal genitalia Normal anal sphincter tone ± Palpable fibrosis along corpus spongiosum ± Enlarged prostate on PR examination	
Medication	Common drugs: Anticholinergics and tricyclic antidepressants Other side effects: Dry mouth, blurred vision, constipation	Onset retention after taking medication	Palpable bladder	

Diagnosis	Background	Key symptoms	Key signs	Additional information
Acute renal failure	Commonly elderly Occurs over hours/days Pre-renal causes: Diarrhoea, hypotension, CCF, nephrotoxins, hepatorenal syndrome Renal causes: Acute tubular necrosis, glomerular disease, vascular disease Post-renal causes: Ureteric obstruction, bladder outlet obstruction	Low urine output <400 millilitres/24 h Nausea/vomiting	Signs vary depending on underlying cause Confusion *Fluid depletion:* Dehydration Postural hypotension No oedema *Or fluid overload:* Raised JVP Peripheral oedema Pulmonary oedema	Emergency medical admission
Phimosis	Non-retractable tight foreskin Can obstruct meatus Infants and young adults Causes: Recurrent balanitis, BXO, trauma, congenital Foreskin does not usually retract before age 2 yrs Often fully retractable by puberty	Poor urine flow Ballooning of foreskin during micturition ± Recurrent balanitis ± Pain on intercourse	Non-retractible foreskin Obstructed meatus	Swelling and erythema of glans penis indicates balanitis
Cauda equina syndrome	Common causes: Lumbar disc herniation, spinal tumour/ trauma, spinal abscess	Acute or gradual onset symptoms Low back pain Pain radiates to one or both legs Difficulty passing or stopping urine Faecal incontinence	Lower limb weakness Lower limb sensory deficit Absent lower limb reflexes Saddle anaesthesia ± Loss of anal tone and sensation	Emergency referral to neurosurgeons Delayed treatment can cause permanent neurological deficit

Chapter 7
Women's Health

Amenorrhoea or oligomenorrhoea

Diagnosis	Background	Key symptoms	Key signs	Additional information
Pregnancy (See Lower abdominal mass)				
Acute stress (See Weight loss)				
Perimenopause/Menopause	Menopause occurs ≈50 yrs age Premature if onset <40 yrs age Preceded by the climacteric Elevated FSH and LH Low oestradiol Symptoms can persist for years	*Climacteric:* Irregular menses (short or long cycles) Menorrhagia Hot flushes Night sweats Palpitations Vaginal dryness Urinary frequency Stress incontinence Low mood or anxiety Insomnia Reduced libido *Menopause:* *As above plus:* Secondary amenorrhoea for ≥12 months	Dry skin Thinning hair Atrophic vaginitis	Risk of osteoporosis, IHD, cerebrovascular disease Post-menopausal bleeding is abnormal if present, refer to exclude endometrial carcinoma
Polycystic ovarian syndrome	Pre-menopausal women Associated with insulin resistance and infertility *≥2 of the following:* Symptomatic Elevated LH (or FSH during menses) and supressed SHBG Polycystic ovaries on ultrasound	Asymptomatic or Irregular or absent menses Excess body hair Frontal balding	± BMI >30 kg/m² ± Acne ± Hirsutism	Weight loss is beneficial
Medication	Common drugs: Parenteral progesterones (e.g. Depo-Provera), Mirena, progesterone-only pill, COCP, cytotoxics Symptoms are often temporary	Onset of amenorrhoea after taking medication	Normal pelvic examination	Exclude pregnancy

Differential Diagnosis in Primary Care, 1st edition. By Nairah Rasul and Mehmood Syed. Published 2009 by Blackwell Publishing, ISBN: 978-1-4051-8036-8

Diagnosis	Background	Key symptoms	Key signs	Additional information
Hyperthyroidism (Thyrotoxicosis)	Primary or secondary Age 20–50 yrs M:F ratio: ≈1:9 Causes: Graves' disease, thyroiditis, toxic nodule, amiodarone Eye changes suggest Graves' disease (e.g. exophthalmos)	Fast palpitations Hyperactivity Sweating Weight loss despite increased appetite Diarrhoea Heat intolerance ± Oligo/amenorrhoea	Tachycardia Lid lag Hair thinning or alopecia Fine postural hand tremor Warm peripheries Gynaecomastia Neck lump Neck lump moves up on swallowing Brisk reflexes ± AF ± Dull percussion over sternum ± Psychosis	Consider thyrotoxic crisis if: Fever Delirium Coma Seizures Jaundice Vomiting
Anorexia nervosa	BMI <17.5 kg/m² Deliberate weight loss Restricted food intake M:F ratio: ≈1:10 Typical onset mid-adolescence Distorted body image Risk factors: Cultural, occupational demands (e.g. modelling, dancing) Associated with: Over-exercise, laxative and diuretic abuse, bulimia	Rapid and severe weight loss "Fear of putting on weight" Low mood Social withdrawal	Bradycardia Hypotension Hypothermia Cachexia Distorted body image Preoccupation with food Depression ± Dental enamel erosion ± Lanugo hair growth	Complications include: Cardiac failure, renal failure, osteoporosis Risk of suicide
Late-onset congenital adrenal hyperplasia	Autosomal recessive Usually 21-hydroxylase deficiency Results in cortisol deficiency and androgen excess Onset late childhood or early adulthood Associated with female infertility and PCOS	May be asymptomatic or Oligomenorrhoea or amenorrhoea Excess hair growth	Precocious puberty Onset ≈8 yrs age in both sexes Acne ± Virilisation ± Hirsutism	
Cushing's syndrome	Causes: Cushing's disease, iatrogenic glucocortoid excess, adrenal tumour, small cell lung carcinoma Commonly 30–50 yrs age M<F Associated with osteoporosis	Increase in abdominal girth Irregular menses or amenorrhoea Excess body hair Easy bruising	Hypertension Moon face Acne Interscapular fat pad (buffalo hump) Purple/red abdominal striae Truncal obesity Thin pigmented skin Hirsutism Proximal muscle weakness	
Hyperprolactinaemia	Causes: Pregnancy, lactation, stress, hypothyroidism, pituitary adenoma, drugs (e.g. phenothiazine, metoclopramide) Prolactin normally under inhibitory dopaminergic control	Oligomenorrhoea or amenorrhoea Breast enlargement Galactorrhoea Reduced libido Infertility Weight gain	Normal secondary sexual characteristics Bilateral milky nipple discharge	Ask about headaches and bitemporal hemianopia
Constitutional delay	Delayed menarche up to 16 yrs age No underlying abnormality Often family history	Primary amenorrhoea	Normal secondary sexual characteritics Normal abdominal examination	Refer for investigation if age >16 yrs
Structural/chromosomal abnormality	Causes include: Genitourinary malformation (e.g. imperforate hymen), testicular feminisation, Turner's syndrome	Primary amenorrhoea	Vary depending on underlying cause ± Normal secondary sexual characteristics	

Bleeding or abdominal pain in pregnancy

Diagnosis	Background	Key symptoms	Key signs	Additional information
Symphysis pubis dysfunction	Over-separation of pubic symphysis Due to increase in ligament laxity Secondary to hormones Common in pregnancy Risk factor: Multiparity	Symptoms are progressive Pain/discomfort in symphysis pubis Radiates to groin, medial thigh, sacroiliac joints Relieved by rest Difficulty walking No history of recent trauma	Tenderness over symphysis pubis Firm pressure on trochanters reproduces pain	Pain can last for years postpartum
Spontaneous abortion/ miscarriage	Fetal death before 24 wks gestation Common in the first trimester Causes: Chromosomal abormality, incompetent cervix, uterine infection, immunological, PCOS Risk factors: Age >35 yrs, drugs, alcohol, smoking	Fresh heavy vaginal bleeding Clots Followed by crampy abdominal pain	Abdomen and uterus non-tender *Incomplete/inevitable miscarriage:* Cervical os open No cervical excitation *Threatened/missed/complete miscarriage:* Cervical os closed No cervical excitation	Very heavy bleeding or a tender uterus warrants immediate admission Consider ectopic pregnancy
Cystitis/Pyelonephritis **See Lower abdominal pain**				
Constipation (See Lower abdominal pain)				
Preterm labour	Onset of labour <37 wks	Painful regular uterine contractions More frequent and longer with time Pink mucous vaginal discharge Amniotic fluid loss	Dilatation and effacement of cervix	Painless irregular uterine contractions (Braxton Hicks) are common in the third trimester
Placenta praevia	Low-lying placenta Minor or major obstruction of cervical os Risk factors: Previous caesarean, multiparity, advancing age Can prevent engagement of fetal head	Acute onset vaginal bleeding (can be profuse) Painless Usually occurs >24 wks	Non-tender uterus Fetal lie often transverse or oblique	Complications include: Severe antepartum haemorrhage and prematurity
Placental abruption	Occurs in the third trimester Risk factors: IUGR, pre-eclampsia, chronic hypertension, smoking, previous history Abruption is concealed or revealed	Acute onset symptoms Constant abdominal pain Frequent uterine contractions ± Vaginal bleeding	Pallor Tachycardia Hypotension Tender hard uterus	Complications include: Fetal death and maternal haemorrhage
Ectopic pregnancy	Occurs in the first trimester Commonest site: Fallopian tube History of positive pregnancy test Common risk factors: PID, IUCD, progesterone-only pill, previous pelvic surgery, advancing age	Acute or chronic onset Unilateral constant iliac fossa pain Followed by dark vaginal bleeding Usually scanty in volume ± History of missed period	Tachycardia Hypotension (in extremis) Lower abdominal rebound tenderness *Pelvic examination:* Cervical excitation Cervical os closed	Emergency gynaecology admission
Appendicitis	Appendix often retrocaecal Commonly 10–20 yrs age Key symptoms often absent in the very young and old	Central colicky abdominal pain Migrates to RIF after hours/days Worse on movement and coughing Becomes progressively worse Anorexia Vomiting	Low-grade fever <39°C Tachycardia Rebound tenderness or guarding in RIF (McBurney's point) Palpation of LIF induces RIF pain (Rovsing's sign) ± Anterior tenderness on PR examination ± Trace haematuria	Consider ectopic pregnancy

Diagnosis	Background	Key symptoms	Key signs	Additional information
Pre-eclampsia	Pregnancy-induced hypertension with proteinuria ± oedema Onset >20 wks gestation Risk factors: Age >40 yrs, first pregnancy ± new partner, multiple pregnancy, obesity, chronic hypertension, family history, renal disease, DM, antiphospholipid antibodies	Often asymptomatic or Epigastric pain Reduced fetal movements Vomiting Frontal headache Visual disturbances (e.g. flashing lights)	BP ≥ diastolic 90 mmHg and/or BP ≥ systolic 160 mmHg Peripheral non-dependent oedema RUQ tenderness Small for gestational age Ankle clonus *Abnormal urinalysis:* ≥1+ Proteinuria ± Fits (Eclampsia) ± Papilloedema	Consider an urgent obstetric review Complications include haemolysis, elevated liver enzymes and low platelets (HELLP Syndrome)
Red degeneration of fibroid	Benign tumour of the myometrium Fibroid grows rapidly Outstrips its blood supply This leads to fibroid haemorrhage Usually occurs in second trimester Often self-limiting	Severe pelvic pain No vaginal bleeding	Fever Localised uterine tenderness	
Hydatiform mole	Trophoblastic tumour invasion of endometrium secretes excess beta-hCG Usually locally invasive Absent viable foetal tissue Can metastasize (choriocarcinoma) Risk factors: Previous history, age >40 yrs, non-Caucasian Associated with: Hyperthyroidism and early pre-eclampsia	History of missed period Positive pregnancy test Vaginal bleeding (can be profuse) Painless Severe vomiting (hyperemesis)	Hypertension Large uterus for dates No foetal heart present	Urgent referral to gynaecology

Breast lump

Diagnosis	Background	Key symptoms	Key signs	Additional information
Benign mammary dysplasia (Cyclical mastalgia)	Normal cyclical breast changes Pre-menopausal women	Symptoms worse premenstrually Breast tenderness and fullness Typically around outer breast Tenderness relieved by menses ± Tender breast lump(s)	Diffuse symmetrical breast nodularity or Ill-defined breast lump Breast tenderness on paplation Lumps become smaller after menses No skin or nipple changes	
Fibroadenoma ("Breast mouse")	Overgrowth of a breast lobule Benign Commonly women age ≤35 yrs Some disappear spontaneously Often recur Regress in menopause Enlarge in pregnancy, HRT, imunosupression	Painless lump Unilateral or bilateral	Solitary or multiple lumps Smooth firm lobulated texture Well-defined margins Diameter usually <3 cm Extremely mobile lump Often get smaller post-menstruation	Usually do not increase in size
Subtype:				
Giant fibroadenoma	Adolescent girls	Rapidly growing lump Painful lump Unilateral or bilateral	Smooth firm lobulated texture Well-defined margins Diameter >3 cm Mobile lump	Refer for excision Unilateral subareolar swelling in prepubescent girls is usually benign
Breast cyst	Middle-aged 35–55 yrs Usually pre-menopausal or on HRT Often benign Multiple cysts increase risk of malignancy Can recur	Acute onset painful lump Unilateral or bilateral	Smooth round or oval lump Well-defined margins Tender on palpation Mobile lump	Cystic carcinomas contain blood and do not disappear post-aspiration

Diagnosis	Background	Key symptoms	Key signs	Additional information
Breast carcinoma	Ductal carcinoma ≈70% Lobular carcinoma ≈20% Other ≈10% M<F Common risk factors: Age >50 yrs, family history, breast cysts, COCP, combined HRT, alcohol, post-menopausal obesity, early menarche or late menopause Metastasizes to lungs, liver, bones, brain	Often painless breast lump Nipple discharge (blood-stained)	Signs usually unilateral Discrete lump Hard irregular texture Fixed to skin or chest Often non-tender on palpation Skin tethering on movement Ipsilateral nipple inversion or discharge ± Skin dimpling (Peau d'orange) ± Axillary LN	Urgent referral for biopsy Scaly itchy eczema confined to the nipple suggests Paget's disease of the nipple
Mammary duct ectasia	Dilatation of major subareolar ducts Due to ductal involution Occasionally become blocked Benign Peri- or post-menopausal women	Symptoms vary and include: Subareolar breast lump Nipple discharge (cheesy/bloody) Non-cyclical breast pain	Unilateral or bilateral Hard tender subareolar lump Nipple inversion	Clinically mimics breast carcinoma, thus refer to exclude malignancy
Fat necrosis	History of breast injury Fat exudes from adipocytes Leads to fibrosis and calcification Benign Lump gradually shrinks with time	Usually painless breast lump	Hard irregular lump Ipsilateral axillary LN ± Localised bruising ± Skin tethering	
Lipoma	Adipose tumour Usually benign Slow growth Commonly adults Often multiple (lipomatosis) Common sites: Neck, trunk, upper arms, shoulders Does not occur on palms or soles Can occur in deeper tissues	Painless lump(s)	Skin-coloured lump Single or multiple Often irregular in shape Usually <5 cm diameter Soft subcutaneous lump Smooth normal skin surface Mobile Not reducible Not pulsatile	If >5 cm and rapid growth, refer to exclude liposarcoma
Galactocele	Ductal milk obstruction Benign Occurs during or post-lactation	Acute onset breast lump Painful	Well-defined lump Smooth texture Tender on palpation Mobile lump	

Breast pain

Diagnosis	Background	Key symptoms	Key signs	Additional information
Benign mammary dysplasia (Cyclical mastalgia)	Normal cyclical breast changes Pre-menopausal women	Symptoms worse premenstrually Breast tenderness and fullness Typically around outer breast Tenderness relieved by menses ± Tender breast lump(s)	Diffuse symmetrical breast nodularity or Ill-defined breast lump Breast tenderness on paplation Lumps become smaller after menses No skin or nipple changes	
Pregnancy	History: Postive pregnancy test, missed period, missed pill, unprotected sex	Amenorrhoea Gradual lower abdominal swelling Breast tenderness Urinary frequency Fatigue ± Nausea/vomiting ± Constipation ± Galactorrhoea	*Palpable uterus:* Suprapubic at 12–14 wks Umbilical ≈20 wks	
Inflamed nipple	Common causes: Chafing during exercise, infection, eczema	Unilateral breast soreness	Apyrexial Local erythema around nipple No palpable breast mass	Scaly itchy eczema confined to the nipple suggests Paget's disease of the nipple

Diagnosis	Background	Key symptoms	Key signs	Additional information
Mastitis	Inflammation and infection of breast tissue Risk factors: Breastfeeding, cracked/sore nipple, nipple piercing	Painful breast swelling	Fever Unilateral breast oedema Erythema and breast tenderness Breast feels hard on palpation Ipsilateral axillary LN ± Purulent nipple discharge	A fluctuant red tender lump indicates an abscess
Breast cyst	Middle-aged 35–55 yrs Usually pre-menopausal or on HRT Often benign Multiple cysts increase risk of malignancy Can recur	Acute onset painful lump Unilateral or bilateral	Smooth round/oval lump Well-defined margins Tender on palpation Mobile lump	Cystic carcinomas contain blood and do not disappear post-aspiration
Galactocele	Ductal milk obstruction Benign Occurs during or post-lactation	Acute onset breast lump Painful lump	Well-defined lump Smooth texture Tender on palpation Mobile lump	
Breast carcinoma	Ductal carcinoma ≈70% Lobular carcinoma ≈20% Other ≈10% M<F Common risk factors: Age >50 yrs, family history, breast cysts, COCP, combined HRT, alcohol, post-menopausal obesity, early menarche or late menopause Metastasizes to lungs, liver, bones, brain	Often painless breast lump Nipple discharge (blood-stained)	Signs usually unilateral Discrete lump Hard irregular texture Fixed to skin or chest Often non-tender on palpation Skin tethering on movement Ipsilateral nipple inversion or discharge ± Skin dimpling (Peau d'orange) ± Axillary LN	Urgent referral for biopsy Scaly itchy eczema confined to the nipple suggests Paget's disease of the nipple
Costochondritis	Idiopathic inflammation of the costal cartilage Commonly affects second costochondral junction Usually self-limiting	Localised chest pain Worse on sneezing, coughing and movement	Unilateral Focal tenderness on palpation ± Costocartilage swelling (Tietze's syndrome)	

Dysmenorrhoea

Diagnosis	Background	Key symptoms	Key signs	Additional information
Primary dysmenorrhoea	No underlying organic pathology Teenagers and young adults Usually improves with age and parity	Symptoms start at onset of menses Lower abdominal cramps ± Radiation to lower back and thighs Lasts ≤3 days ± Breast tenderness ± Vomiting ± Diarrhoea	Normal abdominal examination	
Endometriosis	Chronic condition Growth of ectopic endometrial tissue Oestrogen-dependent Age 30–45 yrs Regresses with pregnancy and menopause Associated with infertility	Often asymptomatic or Secondary dysmenorrhoea Chronic pelvic pain Deep dyspareunia ± Cyclical pain on passing motions	*Pelvic examination:* ± Tenderness in posterior fornix or adnexae ± Adnexal mass	

Diagnosis	Background	Key symptoms	Key signs	Additional information
Pelvic inflammatory disease	Acute or chronic infection Often polymicrobial Risk factors: STIs, IUCD, uterine instrumentation, post-termination, miscarriage Associated with: Subfertility, ectopic pregnancy, chronic pelvic pain	May be asymptomatic or Menorrhagia Bilateral lower abdominal pain Deep dyspareunia Vaginal discharge	Lower abdominal tenderness ± Fever *Pelvic examination:* Bilateral adnexal tenderness Cervical excitation *Speculum examination:* Mucopurulent cervical discharge Cervicitis	Pregnant women should be urgently referred to gynaecology
Intrauterine contraceptive device	Symptoms are usually temporary Common in the first 3 months	Menorrhagia or prolonged bleeding Intermenstrual bleeding Spotting No dyspareunia	Normal abdominal examination Threads present	Complications include: PID (especially within the first 3 wks), ectopic pregnancy, IUCD expulsion
Pelvic congestion syndrome	Dilatation and stasis of pelvic veins Likely due to excess oestrogen Commonly pre-menopausal	Constant lower abdominal pain Dull in nature Relieved by lying down Deep dyspareunia No vaginal discharge	Mild tenderness in iliac fossae ± Bluish discoloration of cervix	

Dyspareunia

Diagnosis	Background	Key symptoms	Key signs	Additional information
Vaginismus	Causes: Fear, pain, history of rape/sexual abuse Associated with: Depression, overwork, drug abuse, relationship problems	Superficial dyspareunia Inability or difficulty in penetration Reduced libido Vaginal dryness Anorgasmia	Tight introitus on PV examinaton Normal pelvic examination	
Vulvovaginitis (See Vaginal discharge)	Any vaginal infection			
Atrophic vaginitis	Post-menopausal women Falling oestrogen levels High vaginal pH Associated with recurrent UTI and vaginal infection	Vaginal or vulval soreness/itch Superficial dyspareunia Post-coital spotting Urgency Dysuria ± Urinary frequency ± Vaginal discharge	Normal abdominal examination Pale dry thin vaginal mucosa ± Contact bleeding ± Mucosal fissures	Significant post-menopausal bleeding warrants further investigation to exclude malignancy
Interstitial cystitis	Chronic relapsing and remitting condition Pancystitis results in bladder fibrosis and contraction Commonly middle-aged women ≈90% have bladder mucosal inflammation and damage (Hunner's ulcers)	Symptoms worse with menstruation Deep dyspareunia Moderate suprapubic or pelvic pain Nocturia Urgency Dysuria No hesitancy	Normal urinalysis	Consider specialist urology referral
Endometriosis	Chronic condition Growth of ectopic endometrial tissue Oestrogen-dependent Age 30–45 yrs Regresses with pregnancy and menopause Associated with infertility	Often asymptomatic or Secondary dysmenorrhoea Chronic pelvic pain Deep dyspareunia ± Cyclical pain on passing motions	*Pelvic examination:* ± Tenderness in posterior fornix or adnexae ± Adnexal mass	

Diagnosis	Background	Key symptoms	Key signs	Additional information
Pelvic inflammatory disease	Acute or chronic infection Often polymicrobial Risk factors: STIs, IUCD, uterine instrumentation, post-termination, miscarriage Associated with: Subfertility, ectopic pregnancy, chronic pelvic pain	May be asymptomatic or Menorrhagia Bilateral lower abdominal pain Deep dyspareunia Vaginal discharge	Lower abdominal tenderness ± Fever *Pelvic examination:* Bilateral adnexal tenderness Cervical excitation *Speculum examination:* Mucopurulent cervical discharge Cervicitis	Pregnant women should be urgently referred to gynaecology
Pelvic adhesions	Causes: Previous pelvic surgery, and/or chronic PID ± History of ectopic pregnancy	Deep dyspareunia Chronic pelvic pain No vaginal discharge ± Infertility	Apyrexial *Pelvic examination:* Bilateral adnexal tenderness	
Pelvic congestion syndrome	Dilatation and stasis of pelvic veins Likely due to excess oestrogen Commonly pre-menopausal	Constant lower abdominal pain Dull in nature Relieved by lying down Deep dyspareunia No vaginal discharge	Mild tenderness in iliac fossae ± Bluish discoloration of cervix	

Irregular vaginal bleeding

Diagnosis	Background	Key symptoms	Key signs	Additional information
Dysfunctional uterine bleeding	Abnormal uterine bleeding No underlying organic pathology A diagnosis of exclusion Commonly adolescents and perimenopausal women Associated with anovulation	Irregular menses or Menorrhagia No history of easy bruising No post-coital bleeding No dyspareunia No vaginal discharge	Normal pelvic examination	Clots indicate excessive blood loss Iron-deficiency anaemia is a common complication
Perimenopause (See Amenorrhoea or oligomenorrhoea)				
Atrophic vaginitis	Post-menopausal women Falling oestrogen levels High vaginal pH Associated with recurrent UTI and vaginal infection	Vaginal or vulval soreness/itch Superficial dyspareunia Post-coital spotting Urgency Dysuria ± Urinary frequency ± Vaginal discharge	Normal abdominal examination Pale dry thin vaginal mucosa ± Contact bleeding ± Mucosal fissures	Significant post-menopausal bleeding warrants further investigation to exclude malignancy
Spontaneous abortion/ miscarriage (See Bleeding or abdominal pain in pregnancy)				
Hormonal breakthrough bleeding	On hormonal contraception or HRT Symptoms can occur in the first few months	Light irregular bleeding or spotting Painless No post-coital bleeding No vaginal discharge	Normal pelvic examination	Exclude: Missed pills, drug interaction, gastroenteritis, pregnancy Persistent bleeding requires further investigation
Ovulation	A peak in mid-luteal progesterone	*Symptoms occur mid-cycle:* Spotting Dull iliac fossa pain (Mittelschmerz) Clear and copious cervical mucus (Spinnbarkheit) Basal body temperature increases by 0.5°C	Normal pelvic examination	

Diagnosis	Background	Key symptoms	Key signs	Additional information
Cervical polyp	Endocervical tumour growth Mostly benign Commonly age 30–50 yrs Can recur Associated with endometrial polyps	Asymptomatic or Intermenstrual bleeding Post-coital spotting Thick whitish vaginal discharge Not offensive	*Speculum examination:* Red/purple polyp Single or multiple Protrudes through cervical os Often <1 cm in size ± Ulceration of polyp surface	All polyps should be removed and biopsied Endometrial polyps can cause menorrhagia
Cervical ectropion (Cervical erosion)	Columnar epithelium of endocervix extends around the external os Oestrogen-dependent Benign Common with puberty, pregnancy, COCP Usually resolves Risk of cervical infection	Usually asymptomatic or Post-coital spotting Mucoid vaginal discharge Not offensive No dyspareunia	*Speculum examination:* Red ring around cervical os	Repeat cervical smear
Cervicitis or vaginitis (See Vaginal discharge)				
Cervical carcinoma	Mostly squamous cell Typical age 30–55 yrs Risk factors: HPV infection, smoking, immunosuppression, promiscuity, unprotected sex, lower social class Cervical intraepithelial neoplasia is pre-cancerous Metastasizes to vagina, uterus, pelvic lymph nodes, rectum, bladder	Intermenstrual bleeding Post-coital bleeding Offensive vaginal discharge	*Speculum examination:* Red or white cervical patches or Cervical mass or ulceration	Refer for urgent colposcopy Cervical smear detects dyskaryosis (CIN) NOT carcinoma

Menorrhagia

Diagnosis	Background	Key symptoms	Key signs	Additional information
Dysfunctional uterine bleeding	Abnormal uterine bleeding No underlying organic pathology A diagnosis of exclusion Commonly adolescents and perimenopausal women Associated with anovulation	Irregular menses or Menorrhagia No history of easy bruising No post-coital bleeding No dyspareunia No vaginal discharge	Normal pelvic examination	Clots indicate excessive blood loss Iron-deficiency anaemia is a common complication
Uterine fibroid (Uterine leiomyoma)	Benign tumour of the myometrium Affects ≈1 in 4 women Usually grow slowly under oestrogen stimulation Vary in size and number Risk factors: Afro-Carribean, perimenopause, family history, nulliparity Regress at menopause unless on HRT	Up to 50% are asymptomatic or Heavy prolonged periods Intermenstrual bleeding Pressure symptoms (e.g. urinary frequency) ± Subfertility	*Pelvic examination:* Enlarged irregular uterus ± Firm pelvic mass	Complications include: Pelvic pain due to fibroid torsion or degeneration Malignancy is rare
Cervical polyp	Endocervical tumour growth Mostly benign Commonly age 30–50 yrs Can recur Associated with endometrial polyps	Asymptomatic or Intermenstrual bleeding Post-coital spotting Thick whitish vaginal discharge Not offensive	*Speculum examination:* Red/purple polyp Single or multiple Protrudes through cervical os Often <1 cm in size ± Ulceration of polyp surface	All polyps should be removed and biopsied Endometrial polyps can cause menorrhagia

Diagnosis	Background	Key symptoms	Key signs	Additional information
Perimenopause/Menopause	Menopause occurs ≈50 yrs age Premature if onset <40 yrs age Preceded by the climacteric Elevated FSH and LH Low oestradiol Symptoms can persist for years	*Climacteric:* Irregular menses (short or long cycles) Hot flushes Night sweats Palpitations Vaginal dryness Urinary frequency Stress incontinence Low mood or anxiety Insomnia Reduced libido *Menopause:* *As above plus:* Secondary amenorrhoea for ≥12 months	Dry skin Thinning hair Atrophic vaginitis	Risk of: Osteoporosis, IHD, cerebrovascular disease Vaginal bleeding post-menopause is abnormal if present, refer to exclude endometrial carcinoma
Acquired hypothyroidism	Age >60 yrs M<F Causes: Autoimmune, thyroiditis, TSH deficiency, postpartum, thyroidectomy, neck radiation, iodine deficiency, drugs (e.g. amiodarone, carbizamole) Associated with: High cholesterol/triglycerides and anaemia	Lethargy Weight gain Constipation Low mood Cold intolerance	Deep hoarse voice Slow cognition (e.g. poor memory) Dry coarse skin Thinning of hair Bradycardia Slow-relaxing tendon reflexes ± Goitre	Beware myxoedema in the elderly: Puffy eyes, hands and feet Cerebellar ataxia Hypothermia Seizures ± Coma
Pelvic inflammatory disease	Acute or chronic infection Often polymicrobial Risk factors: STIs, IUCD, uterine instrumentation, post-termination, miscarriage Associated with: Subfertility, ectopic pregnancy, chronic pelvic pain	May be asymptomatic or Menorrhagia Bilateral lower abdominal pain Deep dyspareunia Vaginal discharge	Lower abdominal tenderness ± Fever *Pelvic examination:* Bilateral adnexal tenderness Cervical excitation *Speculum examination:* Mucopurulent cervical discharge Cervicitis	Pregnant women should be urgently referred to gynaecology
Intrauterine contraceptive device (See Dysmenorrhoea)				
Endometrial hyperplasia (Cystic glandular hyperplasia)	Abnormal endometrial cell proliferation Due to high oestrogen and low progesterone Common risk factors: PCOS, oestrogen therapy, tamoxifen Can be premalignant	Irregular or prolonged menses Intermenstrual bleeding ± Post-menopausal bleeding	Normal pelvic examination	Post-menopausal bleeding is abnormal if present, refer to exclude endometrial carcinoma
Endometrial carcinoma	Usually adenocarcinoma Oestrogen-dependent Typical age >55 yrs Risk factors: Late menopause, obesity, nulliparity, unopposed oestrogen therapy, tamoxifen, family or personal history of breast, ovarian or colon carcinoma Combined HRT and COCP are protective	Post-menopausal bleeding Initially light and intermittent May become heavy and continuous	Normal pelvic examination or pelvic mass in advanced disease	Urgent referral to gynaecology

Nipple discharge

Diagnosis	Background	Key symptoms	Key signs	Additional information
Pregnancy (See Lower abdominal mass)				
Intraduct papilloma	Single or multiple papillomas Multiple papillomatosis is premalignant Commonly pre-menopausal women	Nipple discharge Straw-coloured or blood-stained	Unilateral No eczema of the nipple ± Small tender subareolar nodule	
Mammary duct ectasia	Dilatation of major subareolar ducts Due to ductal involution Occasionally become blocked Benign Peri- or post-menopausal women	Symptoms vary and include: Subareolar breast lump Nipple discharge (cheesy/bloody) Non-cyclical breast pain	Unilateral or bilateral Hard tender subareolar lump Nipple inversion	Clinically mimics breast carcinoma thus refer to exclude malignancy
Mastitis	Inflammation and infection of the breast tissue Risk factors: Breastfeeding, cracked/sore nipple, nipple piercing	Painful breast swelling	Fever Unilateral breast oedema Erythema and breast tenderness Breast feels hard on palpation Ipsilateral axillary LN ± Purulent nipple discharge	A firm red tender lump indicates an abscess
Infected gland of Montgomery	Infected sebaceous gland(s) of the areola Benign Commonly young women Enlarges in pregnancy and lactation Usually resolves spontaneously	Nipple tenderness	Unilateral areolar lump/swelling Normal nipple	
Hyperprolactinaemia	Causes: Pregnancy, lactation, stress, hypothyroidism, pituitary adenoma, drugs (e.g. phenothiazine, metoclopramide) Prolactin normally under inhibitory dopaminergic control	Oligomenorrhoea or amenorrhoea Breast enlargement Galactorrhoea Reduced libido Infertility Weight gain	Normal secondary sexual characteristics Bilateral milky nipple discharge	Ask about headaches and bitemporal hemianopia
Breast carcinoma	Ductal carcinoma ≈70% Lobular carcinoma ≈20% Other ≈10% M<F Common risk factors: Age >50 yrs, family history, breast cysts, COCP, combined HRT, alcohol, post-menopausal obesity, early menarche or late menopause Metastasizes to lungs, liver, bones, brain	Often painless breast lump Nipple discharge (blood-stained)	Signs usually unilateral Discrete lump Hard irregular texture Fixed to skin or chest Often non-tender on palpation Skin tethering on movement Ipsilateral nipple inversion or discharge ± Skin dimpling (Peau d'orange) ± Axillary LN	Urgent referral for biopsy Scaly itchy eczema confined to the nipple suggests Paget's disease of the nipple

Vaginal discharge

Diagnosis	Background	Key symptoms	Key signs	Additional information
Physiological	Onset post-puberty Pre-menopausal women Causes: Menstrual cycle, pregnancy, hormone contraception	Clear or milky discharge Not offensive No vulval soreness or itch	Normal pelvic examination	

Diagnosis	Background	Key symptoms	Key signs	Additional information
Bacterial vaginosis	Deficiency of vaginal *Lactobacilli* Overgrowth of anaerobes, *Gardnerella*, *Mycoplasma hominis* Not sexually transmitted Risk factors: Douching, detergents, raised vaginal pH, smoking, IUCD High recurrence Can resolve without treatment	≈50% are asymptomatic Grey or white thin discharge Fishy odour No vulval soreness or itch	Normal pelvic examination	Complications include: Preterm labour, PID, endometritis
Vaginal candidiasis (Thrush)	Commonly *Candida albicans* Risk factors: Pregnancy, broad-spectrum antibiotics, immunosupression, DM	Thick cheesy discharge Not offensive Vulval soreness and itch Superficial dyspareunia Dysuria No urinary frequency	Inflamed vulva Satellite lesions Normal cervix ± Vulval mucosal fissures	
Chlamydia trachomatis	Sexually transmitted Commonly age <25 yrs Incubation 1–3 wks Risk factors: New sexual partner, unprotected sex, perinatal transmission Associated with PID and infertility	≈80% are asymptomatic Mucopurulent discharge Dyspareunia Dysuria (urethritis) Intermenstrual or post-coital bleeding Lower abdominal pain	Fever Lower abdominal tenderness *Pelvic examination:* Adnexal tenderness Cervical excitation *Speculum examination:* Inflamed cevix ± Contact bleeding Endocervical discharge	Can cause Reiters syndrome: Conjunctivits, urethritis, arthritis Consider referral to GUM clinic for contact tracing
Neiserria gonorrhoea	Sexually transmitted Affects mucous membranes Commonly age <25 yrs Incubation 3–5 days Risk factors: New sexual partner, unprotected sex, perinatal transmission Associated with PID and infertility	≈50% are asymptomatic Mucopurulent discharge Dysuria (urethritis) Intermenstrual or post-coital bleeding Lower abdominal pain Anorectal discomfort (proctitis)	Fever Lower abdominal tenderness ± Pharyngitis *Pelvic examination:* Adnexal tenderness Cervical excitation ± Bartholinitis *Speculum examination:* Endocervical discharge ± Inflamed cervix	Consider referral to GUM clinic for contact tracing Disseminated gonoccocal infection is a rare complication: Fever, rash, septic arthritis, endocarditis, meningitis
Genital herpes	Commonly due to HSV Type I Occasionally HSV Type II via autoinocluation and/or oral sex Typically young adults Usually sexually transmitted Increased risk of acquiring HIV			Asymptomatic individuals can still be infectious Transmission can occur after many years Consider referral to GUM clinic for contact tracing and STI screening
Subtypes:				
Primary HSV	First episode of infection Usually resolves within 4 wks Post-recovery, virus remains dormant in local sensory ganglia	Onset of symptoms ≤1 wk post-infection Flu-like prodrome Lasts up to 7 days Genital tingling Followed by painful genital ulcers Dysuria ± Vaginal discharge	Multiple vesicles or ulcers Heal with crusting Bilateral lesions Tender on palpation Affects cervix and introitus Tender inguinal LN	
Reactivated HSV	Reactivation occurs in ≈75% Usually resolves within 10 days Attacks become less frequent with time	May be asymptomatic or As above but less severe	As above but less severe Lesions often unilateral	

Diagnosis	Background	Key symptoms	Key signs	Additional information
Trichomonas vaginalis	Sexually transmitted Incubation 4 days to 3 wks Risk factors: New sexual partner, unprotected sex	≈50% are asymptomatic Yellow or green frothy discharge Offensive Vulval soreness/itch Superficial dyspareunia Dysuria No urinary frequency	*Speculum examination:* Inflamed vulval or vaginal mucosa Punctate cervical haemorrhages ("Strawberry" cervix)	
Pelvic inflammatory disease	Acute or chronic infection Often polymicrobial Risk factors: STIs, IUCD, uterine instrumentation, post-termination, miscarriage Associated with: Subfertility, ectopic pregnancy, chronic pelvic pain	May be asymptomatic or Bilateral lower abdominal pain Deep dyspareunia Vaginal discharge Menorrhagia Dysmenorrhoea	Lower abdominal tenderness ± Fever *Pelvic examination:* Bilateral adnexal tenderness Cervical excitation *Speculum examination:* Mucopurulent cervical discharge Cervicitis	Pregnant women should be urgently referred to gynaecology
Cervical polyp or ectropion (See Irregular vaginal bleeding)				
Foreign body	Women and children	Offensive vaginal discharge Lower abdominal pain	Foreign body in vagina (e.g. retained tampon)	Beware sexual abuse in children Retained tampon can cause Toxic shock syndrome

Vulval itch

Diagnosis	Background	Key symptoms	Key signs	Additional information
Vaginal candidiasis (Thrush)	Commonly *Candida albicans* Risk factors: Pregnancy, broad-spectrum antibiotics, immunosupression, DM	Thick cheesy discharge Not offensive Vulval soreness and itch Superficial dyspareunia Dysuria No urinary frequency	Inflamed vulva Satellite lesions Normal cervix ± Mucosal fissures	
Genital warts	HPV infection Usually Types 6 and 11 Usually sexually transmitted Risk factors: Smoking, multiple sexual partners, immunosupression Incubation weeks to months Lifelong subclinical infection may persist ≈1/3 resolve spontaneously High recurrence	Painless genital lumps Itchy ± Discharge	Pink or red papules Often multiple May coalesce ("cauliflower") Affects: Introitus, vulva, cervix, perineum	Low risk of malignancy Consider referral to GUM clinic for STI screening
Atrophic vaginitis (See Dyspareunia)				
Chemical dermatitis	Risk factors: Bubble baths, detergents, douches, sanitary wear	No vaginal discharge	Inflamed vulva Normal cervix	
Trichomonas vaginalis	Sexually transmitted Incubation 4 days to 3 wks Risk factors: New sexual partner, unprotected sex	≈50% are asymptomatic Yellow or green frothy discharge Offensive Vulval soreness/itch Superficial dyspareunia Dysuria No frequency	*Speculum examination:* Inflamed vulval/vaginal mucosa Punctate cervical haemorrhages ("Strawberry" cervix)	
Ammoniacal vulvitis	Prolonged skin exposure to urine Risk factors: Immobility, dementia, soiled nappies	Vulval soreness/itch No vaginal discharge	Offensive body odour Inflamed perineum	

Diagnosis	Background	Key symptoms	Key signs	Additional information
Pediculosis pubis (Pubic/crab lice)	Female louse lays eggs Feeds on human blood Egg incubation lasts 8 days Commonly affects adults Usually affects pubic and/or peri-anal hair Spread via close body contact	Itchy pubic hair	Faint blue spots on affected skin Grey or brown lice (2 mm size) Nits (shiny transparent eggs)	
Threadworm	Due to *Enterobius vermicularis* Commonly affects children Faecal–oral spread or inhalation Risk factors: Poor hygiene, overcrowding Eggs laid at night Around anus, vagina, urethra Adult worms live up to 6 wks	Intense itching of anus or vulva Worse at night Disturbed sleep	White cotton-like threads Mobile around anus or vulva *Positive sellotape test:* Early morning application of sellotape to anus demonstrates eggs	
Dermatological condition (See Scales or plaques)	Causes include: Psoriasis, tinea cruris, lichen simplex chronicus			
Vulval carcinoma (See Vulval lump or ulcer)				

Vulval lump or ulcer

Diagnosis	Background	Key symptoms	Key signs	Additional information
Boil (Furuncle)	Deep infection of a hair follicle Usually *Staphylococcus aureus* Common areas: Face, neck, armpits, buttocks, anogenital Usually self-limiting	Painful lump Gradually enlarges	Hard red epidermal nodule Surrounds hair follicle Tender on palpation Fluctuant Mobile ± Pus discharge from centre ± Inguinal LN	Infection of adjacent hair follicles (carbuncle), fever or cellulitis warrants antibiotics
Sebaceous cyst (Epidermoid cyst)	Proliferation of epidermal cells in the dermis Benign Slow growth Commonly young adults M>F Common sites: Face, trunk, neck, extremities, scalp Often resolves spontaneously Usually recurs if not excised	Painless lump(s)	Skin-coloured lump Single or multiple Often round or oval Variable in size Firm subcutaneous nodule Central punctum Fixed to skin Not reducible Not pulsatile ± Uninfected foul cheese-like discharge	A tender and erythematous cyst suggests infection
Genital warts	HPV infection Usually Types 6 and 11 Commonly sexually transmitted Risk factors: Smoking, multiple sexual partners, immunosupression Incubation weeks to months Lifelong subclinical infection may persist ≈1/3 resolve spontaneously High recurrence	Painless genital lumps Itchy ± Discharge	Pink or red papules Often multiple May coalesce ("cauliflower") Affects: Introitus, vulva, cervix, perineum	Low risk of malignancy Consider referral to GUM clinic for STI screening
Vulval carcinoma	Mostly squamous cell Commonly age >60 yrs Risk factors: Squamous dysplasia, HPV, lichen sclerosis, smoking Spreads slowly Metastasizes to groin and pelvic LN	Itchy or painful lump ± Minor bleeding	Papular or warty mass Or irregular ulcer Common areas: Labia majora, clitoris, perineum ± Hard fixed inguinal LN	Persistent ulcers should be referred for biopsy to exclude malignancy

Diagnosis	Background	Key symptoms	Key signs	Additional information
Bartholin's cyst	Blocked gland of the labia minora Usually contains sterile mucus Age 20–30 yrs Risk factors: Nulliparous and low parity	Asymptomatic or Painful lump Superficial dyspareunia Difficulty walking (wide-legged swagger)	Unilateral swelling Fluctuant Affects posterolateral introitus ± Tender on palpation	An acute tender red swelling with fever suggests a Bartholin's abscess
Indirect inguinal hernia (See Groin swelling)				
Genitourinary prolapse	Weak pelvic floor muscles Risk factors: Advancing age, vaginal delivery, obesity, spina bifida Common prolapses: Bladder, urethra, uterus, rectum, vaginal vault, bowel	Vary depending on type of prolapse *Common symptoms:* Dragging sensation or "something coming down" Worse on standing, coughing or straining Urinary symptoms (e.g. frequency, incontinence) Coital difficulty	Vaginal walls bulge on straining or coughing	
Vulval varicosity	Caused by progesterone and increased pelvic weight Benign Commonly occur in pregnancy Usually resolve postpartum	Painful and sore labia Worse on standing Fatigue	*On standing:* Bluish swelling of labia majora	
Urethral caruncle	Fleshy outgrowth of distal urethra Due to distal urethral prolapse Caused by oestrogen deficiency Benign Post-menopausal women	Usually asymptomatic or Dysuria Superficial dyspareunia Minor vaginal bleeding	*Pelvic examination:* Red ring of mucosa around posterior urethral orifice Soft and non-tender on palpation	Exclude UTI
Chancroid	Tropical STI Due to *Haemophilis ducreyi* M>F Incubation 3–10 days Endemic to: Asia, Africa, South America Ulcer occurs at site of contact Does not spread to distant sites Increases risk of HIV transmission	Systemically well Very painful ulcer	Single or multiple genital ulcers Irregular edge Not indurated Necrotic base Purulent discharge Bleeds on contact Tender inguinal LN ± Unilateral buboes (necrotic pus-filled inguinal LN)	Consider referral to GUM clinic for STI screening
Granuloma inguinale	Tropical STI Caused by *Klebsiella granulomatis* M>F Age 20–40 yrs Incubation 8–80 days Endemic to: SE India and South America Spreads slowly Destroys infected tissue	Painless nodules Often affects genitals or anus	Solitary or multiple nodules Beefy red granulomatous texture Gradually enlarges Bursts to form an open ulcer Bleeds on contact Affects: Labia, anus and/or inguinal area Depigmentation of affected skin	Consider referral to GUM clinic for STI screening
Lymphogranuloma venereum	Tropical STI Caused by a *Chlamydia trachomatis* serotype M>F Age 20–40 yrs Endemic to: SE Asia, India, South America, Carribean, Africa			Consider referral to GUM clinic for STI screening
Stages:				
Primary	3 days to 3 wks post-infection More commonly affects men Resolves rapidly	Painless genital ulcer ± Dysuria	Shallow ulcer	

Diagnosis	Background	Key symptoms	Key signs	Additional information
Secondary	Up to several months post-infection	Malaise Arthralgia Nausea/vomiting	Fever Tender inguinal LN Bubo development (necrotic pus-filled inguinal LN) ± Skin rash	
Tertiary	Up to 20 yrs post-infection	Regional pain and bleeding	Regional strictures (e.g. rectal)	
Syphilis	*Treponema pallidum* infection Transmission: Sexual or perinatal Spread via blood and lymphatics			Consider referral to GUM clinic for contact tracing
Stages:				
Primary syphilis	Up to 90 days post-infection Chancre at site of contact Infectious Usually heals within 6 wks	Painless ulcer	Solitary non-tender ulcer (chancre) Round or oval Indurated base and clear discharge Bright-red margin Regional enlarged painless LN	Serological test becomes positive 3–4 wks post-infection
Secondary syphilis	Early latent period <2 yrs post-infection Late latent period >2 yrs post-infection Untreated ≈65% remain asymptomatic	Asymptomatic (latent) or Malaise Myalgia Headaches Non-itchy rash	Latent (absent) signs or Mild fever Generalised painless LN Symmetrical maculopapular rash Affects: Palms, soles, trunk, face Condylomata lata (warts) Affects: Anus and labia	Syphilis may become latent at any stage Symptoms usually abate after a few months
Tertiary syphilis	3–12 yrs post-infection Chronic granulomatous lesions Affects: Bone, skin, mucous membranes, viscera Often cause tissue necrosis	Painless ulcers	Firm red ulcers Can occur anywhere on body	
Quaternary syphilis	>20 yrs post-infection Neurosyphilis and cardiovascular syphilis (e.g. aortic regurgitation)	*General paralysis of insane:* Headaches Poor memory Mood changes *Tabes dorsalis:* Lightning pains in legs Bowel or bladder incontinence Paraesthesia	*General paralysis of insane:* Delusions Confusion Hand tremor *Tabes dorsalis:* Argyll Robertson pupils Ataxia Absent reflexes	Quaternary syphilis is rare
Bechet's disease	Multi-system autoimmune disorder Age 15–45 yrs M>F Associated with HLA-B51	Recurrent symptoms Fatigue Painful mouth and genital ulcers Tender shins Painful eye	Fever Oral and genital ulcers with scarring Erythema nodosum Anterior uveitis ± Symptomatic involvement of other systems (e.g DVT, diarrhoea, arthralgia)	

Chapter 8
Men's Health

Gynaecomastia

Diagnosis	Background	Key symptoms	Key signs	Additional information
Obesity	BMI >30 kg/m² Common risk factors: Family history, inactivity, fatty diet, social deprivation, alcohol abuse Associated with: IHD, hypertension, Type II DM, sleep apnoea, osteoarthritis	Weight gain can be rapid or gradual Breathless on exertion	BMI >30 kg/m² Pseudogynaecomastia No palpable breast tissue behind areola Normal respiratory examination	Pseudoygnaecomastia is diffuse breast enlargement due to excess adipose tissue
Medication	Common drugs: Spironolactone, cimetidine, digoxin, finasteride, marijuana, anabolic steroids, antipsychotics	Onset of gynaecomastia after taking medication	Bilateral gynaecomastia Palpable disc of breast tissue behind areola Firm or rubbery texture Mobile ± Tenderness on palpation	
Puberty	Adolescent breast hypertrophy Increase in oestrogen to androgen ratio Benign Adolescent boys ≈14 yrs age Often regresses within 3 yrs	Breast enlargement	Unilateral or Bilateral asymmetrical gynaecomastia Palpable disc of breast tissue behind areola Firm or rubbery texture Mobile ± Tenderness on palpation	
Lung carcinoma	Incidence increases >40 yrs age Risk factors: Smoking, industrial pollutants (e.g. arsenic, iron oxide, asbestos), radiation	Chronic cough Haemoptysis Chronic breathlessness Chest or shoulder pain Weight loss	Cachexia Anaemia Clubbing Supraclavicular or axillary LN Bilateral gynaecomastia ± Chest signs (e.g. consolidation, effusion) ± Metastases (e.g. bony tenderness, confusion, hepatomegaly)	Histological subtypes: Squamous ≈30% Adenocarcinoma ≈30% Small (oat cell) ≈25% Large cell ≈15% Alveolar cell <1%

Differential Diagnosis in Primary Care, 1st edition. By Nairah Rasul and Mehmood Syed. Published 2009 by Blackwell Publishing, ISBN: 978-1-4051-8036-8

Diagnosis	Background	Key symptoms	Key signs	Additional information
Cirrhosis	Irreversible liver fibrosis and nodule formation M>F Common causes: Alcohol abuse, chronic hepatitis B/C, PBC, Wilson's disease, haemochromatosis, cryptogenic	Symptoms often few or vague Anorexia Gradual weight loss Fatigue	Bruising Clubbing Palmar erythema Dupuytren's contracture Spider naevi above waist Gynaecomastia Dilated peri-umbilical veins Hepatomegaly ± Splenomegaly *Late signs:* Jaundice Ascites Leukonychia Flapping tremor (encephalopathy) Small firm irregular or nodular liver	Complications: Oesophageal varices, ascites, encepalopathy, HCC, heptorenal syndrome Abnormal coagulation is a sensitive test of liver function
Hyperthyroidism (Thyrotoxicosis)	Primary or secondary Age 20–50 yrs M:F ratio: ≈1:9 Causes: Graves' disease, thyroiditis, toxic nodule, amiodarone Eye changes suggest Graves' disease (e.g. exophthalmos)	Fast palpitations Hyperactivity Sweating Weight loss despite increase appetite Diarrhoea Heat intolerance	Tachycardia Lid lag Hair thinning or alopecia Fine postural hand tremor Warm peripheries Gynaecomastia Neck lump Neck lump moves up on swallowing Brisk reflexes ± AF ± Dull percussion over sternum ± Psychosis	Consider thyrotoxic crisis if: Fever Delirium Coma Seizures Jaundice Vomiting
Chronic renal failure	Stage 4 or 5 chronic kidney disease eGFR monitors disease progress Common causes: DM, hypertension, PKD, glomerulonephritis, nephrotoxic drugs (e.g. NSAIDS, aminoglycosides), obstructive uropathy Associated with: IHD, stroke, PVD	Poor concentration Pruritis Fatigue Nausea Anorexia Breathless on exertion ± Oliguria	Hypertension Bilateral gynaecomastia Sallow complexion Anaemia Uraemic fetor Heart failure Pleural effusion Peripheral oedema ± Palpable bladder (in obstruction) *Abnormal urinalysis:* Proteinuria Haematuria	Common endocrine complications: Hypocalcaemia, hyperphosphataemia, secondary hyperparathyroidism, hyperkalaemia
Testicular carcinoma (See Scrotal swelling or pain)				
Hyperprolactinaemia	Prolactin normally under inhibitory dopaminergic control Causes: Stress, hypothyroidism, pituitary adenoma, drugs (e.g. phenothiazine, metoclopramide)	Impotence Galactorrhoea Reduced libido Reduced facial hair	Bilateral gynaecomastia Bilateral milky nipple discharge	Ask about headaches and bilateral temporal hemianopia
Kleinfelter's syndrome	Sex chromosome disorder An extra X chromosome i.e. XXY Derived from either parent Risk factor: Advanced maternal age Associated with: Azoospermia, IHD, IDDM, hypothyroidism, breast carcinoma	Delayed speech or Learning difficulties Loss of libido Impotence	Bilateral gynaecomastia Tall stature Truncal obesity Sparse body and facial hair Small firm testes (hypogonadism) Reduced muscle power	Variant karyotypes include an extra X and Y chromosome and mosaic (only some body cells are affected)

Impotence/erectile dysfunction

Diagnosis	Background	Key symptoms	Key signs	Additional information
Psychological/emotional	Causes: Relationship problems, depression, stress, performance anxiety Increase prevalance with age Usually transient	Acute onset impotence Intermittent episodes Premature or absent ejaculation Morning erection achieved Poor sleep	Normal genital examination Lower-limb pulses present	
Drugs and medication	Common drugs: Beta blockers, antidepressants, antipsychotics, cyproterone acetate, antihistamines, H2 antagonists, recreational drugs (e.g. heroin, amphetamines)	Onset of impotence after taking medication Unable to achieve morning erection	Normal genital examination Lower limb pulses present	
Alcohol abuse	Risk factors: Previous history, family history, binge drinking, poverty, emotional stress, drug addiction, occupation (e.g. publican) Associated with social and mental health problems	Loss of libido Unable to achieve morning erection Poor sleep ± Aggression *Positive CAGE questionnaire*: Wants to Cut down on alcohol Annoyed at being criticised about drinking Feels Guilty about drinking Needs a morning Eye opener	*Acute alcohol withdrawal:* Tachycardia Hypertension Sweating Coarse hand tremor Alcoholic foetor Malnourished ± Delirium tremens ± Cirrhosis	
Physical trauma	Causes include: Pelvic/perineal trauma, spinal fracture, post-operative (e.g. TURP, radical prostatectomy)	Onset of impotence post-trauma	Lower limb pulses present ± Normal genital examination ± Lower limb neuropathy	
Peripheral vascular disease	Atherosclerosis of small and/or large arteries Commonly affects lower limbs Risk factors: Advancing age, smoking, DM, hypertension, hyperlipidaemia, obesity Associated with IHD and stroke	Vary depending on severity *Calf claudication:* Intermittent calf pain Worse on walking Relieved by rest *Rest pain:* Severe leg and forefoot pain Worse at rest (e.g. in bed) Relieved by sitting in a chair or standing *Gangrene:* Patches of blackened lower limb ± Pus (indicates infection)	Loss of lower limb hair Cold limbs on palpation Weak or absent lower limb pulses ± Leg or foot pressure ulcers ± Radio-femoral delay *Positive Buerger's Test:* Bilateral 45° leg raise causes pale feet/legs (ischaemia) followed by reactive hyperaemia when sitting with legs off bed	Always compare right with left Gangrene warrants an emergency vascular opinion
Subtype:				
Leriche syndrome	Bilateral aorto-iliac occlusion	Bilateral buttock claudication Bilateral thigh claudication Gradual onset impotence	As above plus Absent femoral pulses	
Diabetic autonomic neuropathy	Affects parasympathetic system Due to poor glycaemic control Common systems affected: Cardiovascular, genitourinary, gastrointestinal, sweat glands, adrenals, eyes	Insidious onset symptoms Heat intolerance Dizziness or syncope on standing Excess facial sweating Gradual onset impotence Urinary retention (bladder atony) Nocturnal diarrhoea Nausea/vomiting Early satiety Bloating	Resting tachycardia Postural hypotension Argyll-Robertson pupil	Complications include: Silent MI, reduced awareness to hypoglycaemia

Diagnosis	Background	Key symptoms	Key signs	Additional information
Peyronie's disease	Fibrous scar tissue (plaque) in the tunica albuginea Commonly middle-aged men Main risk factor: Penile trauma ≈5% associated with Dupuytren's contracture Can resolve spontaneously	*Symptoms occur on erection:* Penile pain Bending of penis Distortion of penis (e.g. shortening) ± Inadequate penetration	No visible penile deformity when flaccid Palpable fibrosis of penile shaft	
Kleinfelter's syndrome	Sex chromosome disorder An extra X chromosome i.e. XXY Derived from either parent Risk factor: Advanced maternal age Associated with: Azoospermia, IHD, IDDM, hypothyroidism, breast carcinoma	Delayed speech or Learning difficulties Loss of libido Impotence	Bilateral gynaecomastia Tall stature Truncal obesity Sparse body and facial hair Small firm testes (hypogonadism) Reduced muscle power	Variant karyotypes include an extra X and Y chromosome and mosaic (only some body cells are affected)

Penile lump or ulcer

Diagnosis	Background	Key symptoms	Key signs	Additional information
Sebaceous cyst (Epidermoid cyst)	Proliferation of epidermal cells in the dermis Benign Slow growth Commonly young adults M>F Common sites: Face, trunk, neck, extremities, scalp Often resolves spontaneously Usually recurs if not excised	Painless lump(s)	Skin-coloured lump Single or multiple lumps Often round or oval Variable in size Firm subcutaneous nodule Central punctum Fixed to skin Not reducible Not pulsatile ± Uninfected foul cheese-like discharge	A tender and erythematous cyst suggests infection
Genital warts	HPV infection Usually Types 6 and 11 Commonly sexually transmitted Risk factors: Smoking, multiple sex partners, immunosupression Incubation weeks to months Lifelong subclinical infection may persist ≈1/3 resolve spontaneously High recurrence	Painless genital lumps Itchy ± Discharge	Pink or red papules Often multiple May coalesce ("cauliflower") Affects: Penile shaft, glans, urethral meatus, perianal	Low risk of malignancy Consider referral to GUM clinic for STI screening
Genital herpes	Commonly due to HSV Type I Occasionally HSV Type II via autoinocluation and/or oral sex Typically young adults Usually sexually transmitted Increased risk of acquiring HIV			Asymptomatic individuals can still be infectious Transmission can occur after many years Consider referral to GUM clinic for contact tracing and STI screening
Subtypes:				
Primary HSV	First episode of infection Usually resolves within 4 wks Post-recovery, virus remains dormant in local sensory ganglia	Onset of symptoms ≤1 wk post-infection Flu-like prodrome Lasts up to 7 days Genital tingling Followed by painful genital ulcers Dysuria ± Rectal or urethral discharge	Multiple vesicles or ulcers Heals with crusting Bilateral lesions Tender Affects: Urethra, penile shaft, anorectal area Tender inguinal LN	Severe pain can cause urinary retention and/or constipation
Reactivated HSV	Reactivation occurs in ≈75% Usually resolves within 10 days Attacks become less frequent with time	May be asymptomatic or As above but less severe	As above but less severe Lesions often unilateral	

Diagnosis	Background	Key symptoms	Key signs	Additional information
Balanitis	Acute inflammation of glans penis ± Foreskin (Balanoposthitis) Commonly young boys and elderly Causes: Fungal/bacterial infection (including STI), skin disorder (e.g. lichen planus), severe oedema, trauma, phimosis, allergy Risk factors: DM, broad spectrum antibiotics, poor hygiene, immunosupression, RVF	Soreness at the end of the penis Dysuria ± Purulent discharge beneath foreskin	Swelling and erythema of glans and/or foreskin Inguinal LN ± Phimosis (in recurrent balanitis)	Exlude DM in recurrent candidal infection
Trauma	Usually involves foreskin Causes include: Zipper, inappropriate foreskin retraction, bites	History of recent trauma Onset penile pain post-trauma ± Bleeding ± Dysuria	Laceration or abrasion of foreskin/penis	
Balanitis xerotica obliterans	Chronic progressive condition Likely a form of lichen sclerosis Causes urethral obstruction Commonly young adults Affects: Foreskin and/or glans penis	Sore itchy glans and/or foreskin Poor urine stream	Atrophic white patches on glans and/or foreskin Shrunken white foreskin Pinhole meatal orifice ± Phimosis	
Reiters syndrome	Sexually or GI related Can be chronic or recurrent M:F ratio. ≈20:1 Age 16–35 yrs Genital causes: *Chlamydia trachomatis, Neiserria gonnorrhoea* Enteric causes: *Campylobacter, Salmonella, Shigella, Yersinia* >60% are HLA-B27 positive Associated with ankylosing spondylitis	Malaise Chronic lower limb large joint pain Dysuria ± Urethral discharge	*Triad signs:* Bilateral conjunctivitis Non-specific urethritis (if sexually related) Mono or polyarthritis (e.g. knees, ankles) ± Fever ± Cachexia ± Balanitis ± Brown aseptic abscesses on soles/palms (Keratoderma blenorrhagica)	Arthritis is seronegative and erosive
Chemical dermatitis	Causes: Poor hygiene, soaps, detergents, overscrubbing, condoms, spermicides, lubricants	Systemically well Sore and itchy penis	Excoriated and inflamed penis	Other body parts may be affected
Chancroid	Tropical STI Due to *Haemophilis ducreyi* M>F Incubation 3–10 days Endemic to: Asia, Africa, South America Ulcer occurs at site of contact Does not spread to distant sites Increases risk of HIV transmission	Systemically well Very painful ulcer	Single or multiple genital ulcers Irregular edge Not indurated Necrotic base Purulent discharge Bleeds on contact Tender inguinal LN ± Unilateral buboes (necrotic pus filled inguinal LN)	Consider referral to GUM clinic for STI screening
Granuloma inguinale	Tropical STI Caused by *Klebsiella granulomatis* M>F Age 20–40 yrs Incubation 8–80 days Endemic to: SE India and South America Spreads slowly Destroys infected tissue	Painless nodules Often affects genitals or anus	Solitary or multiple nodules Beefy red granulomatous texture Gradually enlarges Bursts to form an open ulcer Bleeds on contact Affects: Penile shaft, anus and/or inguinal area Depigmentation of affected skin	Consider referral to GUM clinic for STI screening

Diagnosis	Background	Key symptoms	Key signs	Additional information
Lymphogranuloma venereum	Tropical STI Caused by a *Chlamydia trachomatis serotype* M>F Age 20–40 yrs Endemic to: SE Asia, India, South America, Carribean, Africa			Consider referral to GUM clinic for STI screening
Stages:				
Primary	3 days to 3 wks post-infection More commonly affects men Resolves rapidly	Painless genital ulcer ± Dysuria	Shallow ulcer	
Secondary	Up to several months post-infection	Malaise Arthralgia Nausea/vomiting	Fever Tender inguinal LN Bubo development (necrotic pus filled inguinal LN) ± Skin rash	
Tertiary	Up to 20 yrs post-infection	Regional pain and bleeding	Regional strictures (e.g. rectal)	
Syphilis	*Treponema pallidum infection* Transmission: Sexual or perinatal Spread via blood and lymphatics			Consider referral to GUM clinic for contact tracing
Stages:				
Primary syphilis	Up to 90 days post-infection Chancre at site of contact Infectious Usually heals within 6 wks	Painless ulcer	Solitary non-tender ulcer (chancre) Round or oval Indurated base and clear discharge Bright red margin Regional enlarged painless LN	Serological test becomes positive 3–4 wks post-infection
Secondary syphilis	Early latent period <2 yrs infection Late latent period >2 yrs infection Untreated ≈65% remain asymptomatic	Asymptomatic (latent) or Malaise Myalgia Headaches Non-itchy rash	Latent (absent) signs or Mild fever Generalised painless LN Symmetrical maculopapular rash Affects: Palms, soles, trunk, face Condylomata lata (warts) Affects anus	Syphilis may become latent at any stage Symptoms usually abate after a few months
Tertiary syphilis	3–12 yrs post-infection Chronic granulomatous lesions Affect bone, skin, mucous membranes, viscera Often cause tissue necrosis	Painless ulcers	Firm red ulcers Can occur anywhere on body	
Quaternary syphilis	>20 yrs post-infection Neurosyphilis and cardiovascular syphilis (e.g. aortic regurgitation)	*General paralysis of insane:* Headaches Poor memory Mood changes *Tabes dorsalis:* Lightning pains in legs Bowel or bladder incontinence Paraesthesia	*General paralysis of insane:* Delusions Confusion Hand tremor *Tabes dorsalis:* Argyll-Robertson pupils Ataxia Absent reflexes	Quaternary syphilis is rare
Bechet's disease	Multi-system autoimmune disorder Age 15–45 yrs M>F Associated with HLA-B51	Recurrent symptoms Fatigue Painful mouth and genital ulcers Tender shins Painful eye	Fever Oral and genital ulcers with scarring Erythema nodosum Anterior uveitis ± Symptomatic involvement of other systems (e.g DVT, diarrhoea, arthralgia)	

Diagnosis	Background	Key symptoms	Key signs	Additional information
Penile carcinoma	Commonly squamous cell Originates in glans or foreskin Typically elderly men Risk factors: Erythroplasia Queyrat, Bowens disease, HPV, BXO, poor hygiene, smoking, chemical exposure (e.g. insecticides, fertilisers) Metastasizes to penile shaft and inguinal LN Early circumcision and personal hygiene may be preventative	Itching or burning beneath foreskin	Solitary lesion on glans or foreskin Indurated ulcer or mass Progressively enlarging Offensive discharge (purulent or blood-stained) Non-tender inguinal LN ± Phimosis	Urgent urology referral

Scrotal swelling or pain

Diagnosis	Background	Key symptoms	Key signs	Additional information
Indirect inguinal hernia (See Groin swelling)				
Sebaceous cyst (Epidermoid cyst)	Proliferation of epidermal cells in the dermis Benign Slow growth Commonly young adults M>F Common sites: Face, trunk, neck, extremities, scalp Often resolves spontaneously Often recur if not excised	Painless lump(s)	Skin-coloured lump Single or multiple Often round or oval Variable in size Firm subcutaneous nodule Central punctum Fixed to skin Not reducible Not pulsatile ± Uninfected foul cheese-like discharge	A tender and erythematous cyst suggests infection
Epididymal cyst	Extratesticular cyst of epididymis Benign Age >40 yrs	Painless scrotal lump	May be solitary or multiple Unilateral or bilateral Smooth texture Lies posterior to and above testis Able to palpate above lump(s) Fluctuant Transluminates Testicle palpable separate from cysts	
Hydrocele	Fluid in the tunica vaginalis Surrounds the testicle			
Subtypes:				
Congenital hydrocele	Processus vaginalis remains patent Communicates with peritoneal fluid Typically benign Underlying pathology rarely present Usually resolves spontaneously by age 1 yr	Painless scrotal swelling Worse on sitting Relieved by lying	Unilateral or bilateral Large testicular swelling Smooth and soft texture Able to palpate above swelling Fluctuant Transluminates Testicle usually not palpable	Urology referral if an inguinal hernia co-exists or hydrocele persists beyond age 1 yr
Adult hydrocele	Underlying pathology usually present Causes: Inflammation, malignancy, trauma, chronic torsion	Painless scrotal swelling Persistent swelling	Unilateral or bilateral Smooth soft testicular swelling Able to palpate above swelling Fluctuant Transluminates Testicle usually not palpable	Refer for ultrasound to exclude underlying malignancy

Diagnosis	Background	Key symptoms	Key signs	Additional information
Varicocele	Dilated veins of the pampiniform plexus in the spermatic cord Affects left testicle > right testicle Commonly adolescents and young adults Associated with male subfertility Left varicocele rarely associated with left renal carcinoma	Dull dragging sensation in testicle Worse at the end of the day	Usually unilateral Varicocele varies in size *On standing:* ± Visible swelling above testicle Spermatic cord feels like "a bag of worms" Non-tender on palpation *On lying down:* Cord swelling may disappear Palpable cough impulse	A varicocele can cause testicular atrophy in adolescents so consider referral
Epididymo-orchitis	Testicular and epididymal infection Causes include: *Mumps, Neisseria gonorrhoea, Chlamydia trachomatis*, coliforms, scrotal trauma, obstructive uropathy (e.g. BPH), Behcet's disease	Acute onset symptoms Scrotal swelling and pain Malaise ± Urethral discharge (in STI) ± Dysuria and frequency (in UTI)	Fever Usually unilateral Scrotal oedema and erythema Tender swollen testicle and epididymis Able to palpate above swelling Does not transluminate Inguinal LN *Positive Prehn's sign:* Scrotal elevation relieves pain	If testicular torsion suspected, seek an urgent urology opinion
Testicular carcinoma	>95% are germ cell tumours of the seminiferous tubules *Germ cell types:* ≈50% Teratomas ≈45% Seminomas ≈5% Yolk sac tumours Age 20–35 yrs Risk factors: Cryptorchidism, family history, low sperm count, Kleinfelter's syndrome Lymphatic spread Primarily to para-aortic LN	Painless lump in testicle Dull dragging sensation in testicle	Irregular lump arising from testicle Heavy and firm texture Typically non-tender Insensitive to palpation Absent inguinal LN ± Hydrocele ± Gynaecomastia ± Left supraclavicular LN (Virchow's node)	Urgent urology referral
Torsion of the testis	Torsion of the spermatic cord Commonly teenagers Risk of torsion in contralateral testis	Acute onset severe testicular pain Usually during physical activity Lower abdominal pain Nausea/vomiting Discomfort on walking ± History of previous testicular pain	Unilateral Scrotal erythema Extremely tender swollen testicle Testicle lies high and horizontal *Negative Prehn's sign:* Scrotal elevation increases pain	Complications: Testicular ischaemia and infarction Warrants emergency urological exploration
Scrotal oedema	Typically elderly Often due to right ventricular failure	Gradual onset scrotal oedema Chronic breathlessness Nausea Anorexia Fatigue	Raised JVP Bilateral scrotal swelling Non-tender testes Leg and sacral pitting oedema Ascites Hepatomegaly (may be pulsatile) ± Cyanosis ± Mild jaundice	Scrotal erythema and tenderness suggests cellulitis

Urethral discharge

Diagnosis	Background	Key symptoms	Key signs	Additional information
Neiserria gonorrhoea	Sexually transmitted Affects mucous membranes Commonly age <25 yrs Incubation 3–5 days Risk factors: New sexual partner, unprotected sex, perinatal transmission Associated with PID and infertility in females	Up to 10% are asymptomatic Purulent urethral discharge Dysuria Urinary frequency	Meatal oedema and erythema ± Epididymo-orchitis ± Acute prostatitis	Consider referral to GUM clinic for contact tracing and STI screening Disseminated gonoccocal infection is a rare complication: Fever, rash, septic arthritis, endocarditis, meningitis

Diagnosis	Background	Key symptoms	Key signs	Additional information
Chlamydia trachomatis	Sexually transmitted Commonly age <25 yrs Incubation 1–3 wks Risk factors: New sexual partner, unprotected sex, perinatal transmission Associated with PID and infertility in females	≈50% are asymptomatic Yellow urethral discharge Dysuria ± Anorectal discomfort (proctitis)	± Fever ± Epididymo-orchitis ± Acute prostatitis	Can cause Reiters syndrome: Conjunctivits, urethritis, arthritis Consider referral to GUM clinic for contact tracing and STI screening
Trichomonas vaginalis	Sexually transmitted Incubation 4 days to 4 wks Risk factors: New sexual partner, unprotected sex	≈50% are asymptomatic Mild urethral discharge Clear or grey discharge Dysuria	Often normal genital examination ± Meatal erythema	Consider referral to GUM clinic for contact tracing and STI screening
Ureaplasma urealyticum	Mycoplasmal bacterium Commensal of lower urogenital tract in the sexually active Causes non-gonococcal urethritis in men and women Transmission: Sexual and perinatal	May be asymptomatic or Urethral discharge, worse in the morning Mild dysuria Meatal irritation	Often normal genital examination ± Meatal erythema	Consider if urethritis is persistent despite treatment
Non-gonoccocal urethritis (Non-specific urethritis)	Common causes: *Chlamydia trachomatis, Ureaplasma urealyticum, Mycoplasma genitalium, Trichomonas vaginalis, idiopathic* Typical age <40 yrs Risk factors: New sexual partner, unprotected sex, anal sex Females tend to be asymptomatic	White urethral discharge Worse in the morning Mild dysuria Urinary frequency Meatal irritation or pruritus	Often normal genital examination *Abnormal urinalysis:* Leucocytes ± Haematuria	Consider referral to GUM clinic for contact tracing and STI screening Complications include: Epididymitis and/or orchitis, prostatitis, Reiter's syndrome

Chapter 9
Musculoskeletal

Ankle pain

Diagnosis	Background	Key symptoms	Key signs	Additional information
Ankle sprain	Ligamental injury History of forced eversion or inversion Usually heals within days to weeks	Painful swollen ankle	Non-tender over malleoli ± Soft tissue swelling and bruising Able to weight bear	Exclude fracture and ligamental tears
Osteoarthritis of the ankle	Degenerative joint disease Risk factors: Advancing age, family history, previous ankle injury, obesity	Ankle pain Worse with activity Relieved by rest Joint stiffness <30 mins in morning or after rest	Systemically well Antalgic gait Reduced ROM of ankle Pain on dorsiflexion Joint swelling and effusion Periarticular tenderness Crepitus Bony swelling and deformity Joint instability	
Achilles tendonitis	Commonly in athletes who over-pronate their feet Risk factors: Unaccustomed exercise with boots, change in playing surface, high exercise intensity	Discomfort on walking or exercise Pain and swelling proximal to insertion of the Achilles tendon	Tender over insertion of Achilles Pain on passive plantar flexion and dorsiflexion Able to lift affected heel from floor when standing on tiptoe	Some drugs can cause Achilles tendon inflammation and predispose to rupture (e.g. steroid, quinolone antibiotics or statins)
Ankle fracture (Pott's fracture)	History of trauma or increased activity Commonly forced ankle inversion	Acute onset ankle pain Rapid swelling and bruising of ankle	*Ottawa rules (indicate X-ray) if:* Unable to weight-bear 4 steps Pain in the malleolar region Bony tenderness at posterior or tip of lateral/medial malleolus ± Ankle deformity	Consider co-existing foot fractures
Ankle ligament tears	History of trauma or fall with inversion of ankle	Acute onset pain Swelling and bruising of ankle Instability of ankle	Tender over lateral malleolus Pronounced inversion or eversion of ankle on passive movement ± Pain on ankle dorsiflexion (if inferior tibulo-fibular ligament damaged)	
Tibialis posterior dysfunction	Ankle pain and dysfunction Causes: Tenosynovitis, longitudinal tears, rupture of tibialis posterior tendon	Discomfort on walking or exercise Pain and swelling of ankle Pain extends from behind medial malleolus to insertion at navicular	Absent arch on heel inversion Painful flat foot Pain on standing on tiptoe on affected foot	
Ruptured Achilles tendon	Commonly athletes May follow unaccustomed exercise Risk factors: Chronic achilles tendonitis, steroid, quinolone antibiotic or statin use	Acute onset pain in posterior ankle Worse during activity Feels like "blow to the ankle" Rapid swelling of ankle post-injury	Antalgic gait Palpable gap in tendon Full plantarflexion of foot possible Unable to lift affected heel from floor when standing on tiptoe	Refer to orthopaedics for surgical repair or immobilisation

Differential Diagnosis in Primary Care, 1st edition. By Nairah Rasul and Mehmood Syed. Published 2009 by Blackwell Publishing, ISBN: 978-1-4051-8036-8

Back pain

Diagnosis	Background	Key symptoms	Key signs	Additional information
Mechanical back pain	Age 20–55 yrs >90% present with low back pain Pain arises from ligaments, discs, facet joints Unnecessary to differentiate exact cause High recurrence Associated with depression	Pain in lower back, lateral thigh or buttock Back pain > limb pain Pain varies between and during episodes Pain worse with certain postures	Normal neurological examination Normal straight leg raise No bony tenderness	Exclude depression and red flags Red flags: Age <20 yrs or >55 yrs Abnormal neurology Thoracic pain Weight loss Fever History of malignancy Use of systemic steroids
Prolapsed lumbar disc	Prolapse of nucleus pulposus Impinges on lumbar nerve roots Age 20–50 yrs Associated with sciatica	Low back pain Radiates to foot or toes Unilateral leg pain > low back pain	Paraesthesia in distribution of pain Straight leg raise induces pain Focal neurology limited to one nerve root	
Vertebral fracture	History of major back trauma Or minor trauma in pathological bones Consider pathological fracture if: History of malignancy, osteoporosis, steroid use, weight loss, thoracic pain, systemic upset	Acute onset back pain Constant pain Worse on lying supine New onset deformity of spine	Loss of height Bony tenderness Palpable vertebral step New kyphosis or scoliosis	Refer for X-ray
Acute pyelonephritis (See Lower abdominal pain)				
Ureteric obstruction (See Lower abdominal pain)				
Prostatitis (See Frequency)				
Vertebral body/disc infection	Infection of a vertebral body or intervertebral disc Commonly i.v. drug users and immunosuppressed Causes include: TB and staphylococci	Severe pain in lower back Worse with rest Relieved by movement Malaise	Fever Tender over intervertebral disc or vertebral body Palpable warmth ± Erythema of overlying skin ± Kyphosis in vertebral collapse ± Groin abscess ± Lower-limb neurology	Emergency admission
Malignancy	Previous history of malignancy Common primary tumours: Breast, lung, prostate Primary bone cancer is rare	Back, rib or hip pain Worse at night Weight loss Malaise *Symptoms of hypercalcaemia:* Lethargy Low mood Polyuria Polydipsia Constipation Muscle weakness	Bony tenderness Occasional soft tissue masses Gradual progressive neuropathy Hepatomegaly Pathological fractures	
Multiple myeloma	Malignant plasma cell proliferation Bone marrow infiltration Bone destruction and marrow failure Commonly age >50 yrs M>F Associated with: Urinary Bence Jones proteins and serum monoclonal protein (e.g. IgG)	Bone pain (typically back, femur, pelvis) Lethargy Anorexia Bruising *Symptoms of hypercalcaemia:* Lethargy Low mood Polyuria Polydipsia Constipation Muscle weakness	Anaemia Bony tenderness Pathological fractures ± Spinal cord/nerve root compression	Complications include: Hyperviscosity, amyloidosis, renal failure Urgent referral to haematology

Diagnosis	Background	Key symptoms	Key signs	Additional information
Paget's disease of the bone	Abnormal osteoclast activity Disorganised bone remodelling Results in larger and weaker bones Age >40 yrs M>F Commonly affects spine, skull and long bones ≈1% cases develop sarcoma	Often asymptomatic or Dull bony pain (e.g. backache) Worse on weight bearing Progressive bone deformity Deafness	Bowing of tibia, femur and/or forearm Frontal bossing Deafness (CN VIII compression) Pathological fractures (e.g. femur)	
Ankylosing spondylitis	Seronegative spondyloarthopathy Facet joint and sacro-iliac joint inflammation Results in spinal fusion Age 18–40 yrs M>F Caucasian predominance ≈90% HLA-B27 positive Positive family history	Low back pain Progressively worse over months Gradually involves thoracic spine Early morning back stiffness Relieved by activity	Reduced spinal movements Lumbar lordosis persists on forward flexion Pain over iliac crests Reduced chest expansion <5 cm *Extra-articular signs:* Inflamed swelling at insertion of Achille's tendon Anterior uveitis Aortic regurgitation Pulmonary fibrosis	
Dissecting abdominal aortic aneurysm (See Upper abdominal mass)				
Lumbar cord compression	Common causes: Trauma, malignancy, prolapsed intervertebral disc *above* L1 level	Acute or gradual onset symptoms Paraesthesia in legs or perineum Difficulty passing or stopping urine Faecal incontinence	Tender lumbar vertebrae Lower limb weakness Lower limb sensory deficit Saddle anaesthesia *UMN signs in lower limbs:* Spasticity Hyperreflexia below level of lesion Upgoing plantars ± Loss of anal tone and sensation	Refer for emergency admission Delayed treatment can cause permanent neurological deficit
Lumbar spondylolisthesis	Displacement of vertebral body on the one below Displacement is typically forwards Commonly involves L4/5 or L5/S1 Causes: Spondylosis due to stress fracture, dysplasia of lumbosacral joints, OA degeneration Commonly athletes and gymnasts	Children usually asymptomatic *Adolescent or adult symptoms:* Chronic backache Radiates to buttocks Worse after standing and exertion ± Sciatica	*Signs in children:* Enhanced lordosis Waddled gait *Adolescent or adult signs:* Flattened buttocks due to disuse Significant transverse loin creases Visible or palpable vertebral step ± Limited straight leg raise (if sciatica) ± Reduced ROM of spine	
Spinal stenosis	Narrowing of the spinal canal Due to hypertrophy at the posterior disc margin and facet joints Commonly >60 yrs age Causes: Chronic disc degeneration and OA	Aching of lower limbs Numbness and paraesthesia in lower limbs Symptoms worse on standing or walking for 10 mins Relieved by sitting or squatting against a wall to flex spine	*At rest:* Normal straight leg raise Normal lower limb pulses No focal neurology *Post-exertion:* Often unilateral signs Focal neurological signs in lower limbs	Unlike claudication, pain is not relieved by standing still
Cauda equina syndrome	Common causes: Lumbar disc prolapse, spinal tumour or trauma, spinal abscess	Acute or gradual onset symptoms Low back pain Pain radiates to one or both legs Difficulty passing or stopping urine Faecal incontinence	Lower limb weakness Lower limb sensory deficit Absent lower limb reflexes Saddle anaesthesia ± Loss of anal tone	Refer for emergency admission Delayed treatment can cause permanent neurological deficit

Calf pain

Diagnosis	Background	Key symptoms	Key signs	Additional information
Cellulitis	Infection of dermis and subcutaneous tissue Commonly streptococcal or staphylococcal infection	Pain over affected areas Spreading erythema and swelling ± Malaise	Well-demarcated erythema Localised warmth and swelling Rapid progression ± Fever	Skin crepitus indicates anaerobic infection Risk of skin necrosis if untreated
Sciatica	Pain in the distribution of the Sciatic nerve Common causes: Lumbar disc prolapse, inflammation, spinal stenosis, malignancy, Paget's , ankylosing spondylitis, vertebral fracture or infection, trauma Most recover within 4 wks of conservative management	Sharp localised pain in buttock Radiates down leg to foot or toes Numbness and paraesthesia Symptoms worse with coughing, sneezing	Normal lower limb pulses *Lasegue test:* Passive straight leg raise limited to ≈30°–80° due to pain Further foot dorsiflexion increases pain Relieved by knee flexion ± *Focal neurology:* Weak foot dorsiflexion (L4/5) Weak great toe dorsiflexion (L5) Reduced sensation in lateral lower leg, dorsum and sole of foot	Exclude bowel and bladder dysfunction
Leg cramps	Commonly affects elderly	Painful muscle spasm in calf Typically occurs at night Worse after exercise	Normal leg examination	
Peripheral vascular disease	Atherosclerosis of small and/or large arteries Commonly affects lower limbs Risk factors: Advancing age, smoking, DM, hypertension, hyperlipidaemia, obesity Associated with IHD, stroke, impotence	Vary depending on severity *Calf claudication:* Intermittent calf pain Worse on walking Relieved by rest *Rest pain:* Severe leg and forefoot pain Worse at rest (e.g. in bed) Relieved by sitting in a chair or standing *Gangrene:* Patches of blackened lower limb ± Pus (indicates infection)	Loss of lower limb hair Cold limbs on palpation Weak or absent lower limb pulses ± Leg or foot pressure ulcers ± Radio-femoral delay *Positive Buerger's Test:* Bilateral 45° leg raise causes pale feet/legs (ischaemia) followed by reactive hyperaemia when sitting with legs off bed	Always compare right with left Gangrene warrants an emergency vascular opinion
Subtype:				
Leriche syndrome	Bilateral aorto-iliac occlusion	Bilateral buttock claudication Bilateral thigh claudication Gradual onset impotence	As above plus Absent femoral pulses	
Superficial thrombophlebitis	Inflammatory response to thrombosis in a superficial vein Commonly age >60 yrs M<F Risk factors: Obesity, thrombophilia, malignancy, smoking, COCP, pregnancy, varicose veins	Localised pain over a vein	Tender vein Bruising around vein Palpable cord-like thickening of vein Localised swelling and erythema	Recurrent thrombophlebitis in different sites (migratory thrombophlebitis) requires investigation to exclude malignancy
Deep vein thrombosis	M<F Risk factors: Trauma or surgery, advancing age, obesity, smoking, long-haul flight, immobility, pregnancy, HRT, COCP, malignancy	Diffuse pain in calf Swelling of calf and ankle	Low-grade fever <39°C Tachycardia Diffuse erythema Venous dilatation Lower leg swelling Tender calf muscle *Homan's sign:* Increased pain on dorsiflexion of foot	Consider PE if chest pain or SOB
Ruptured Baker's cyst	Synovial sac of knee joint herniates into popliteal fossa Ruptures causing leakage of synovial fluid into calf Risk factor: Arthritic knee	Diffuse pain in calf Swelling of calf and ankle	Diffuse erythema Lower leg swelling Tender calf muscle *Homan's sign:* Increased pain on dorsiflexion of foot	Mimics DVT which may also co-exist

Diagnosis	Background	Key symptoms	Key signs	Additional information
Cauda equina syndrome (See Back pain)				
Compartment syndrome	Oedema in an osteofascial compartment Causes increased pressure and ischaemia of affected limb Risk factors: Limb injury, tight plaster cast	Painful limb Numbness Weakness Symptoms worse with activity	Pale or cyanotic limb Swollen limb Weak peripheral pulse Reduced sensation Reduced power in distal muscles Passive extension of fingers or toes increases pain	A palpable pulse does not exclude diagnosis

Elbow pain

Diagnosis	Background	Key symptoms	Key signs	Additional information
Lateral epicondylitis (Tennis elbow)	Caused by repeated strain on the common extensor tendon	Gradual onset pain Radiates to forearm and lateral side of elbow	Usually unilateral Tender lateral epicondyle Pain on resisted wrist extension (e.g. opening jar)	
Medial epicondylitis (Golfer's elbow)	Caused by repeated strain on the common flexor tendon	Gradual onset pain Radiates to forearm and medial side of elbow ± Paraesthesia of 4th/5th fingers	Usually unilateral Tender medial epicondyle Pain on resisted wrist pronation (e.g. shaking hands)	
Olecranon bursitis	Common causes: Elbow pressure, recurrent minor trauma, gout, infection, RA	Pain and swelling over olecranon	Red boggy swelling over olecranon Tenderness on palpation Full ROM of elbow	Aspirate fluid to exclude sepsis
Pulled elbow	Traction injury to elbow causes subluxation of radial head (e.g. pulling child up by the hand) Age <5 yrs M>F Commonly left arm > right arm	Pain over the forearm and elbow Child does not use arm	Pain over radial head	Immediate recovery on reduction
Osteoarthritis of the elbow	Degenerative joint disease Common causes: Intra-articular fractures, loose bodies, crystal deposition disorders (e.g. gout)	Mild elbow pain Worse with activity Relieved by rest Joint stiffness worse after rest	Systemically well Enlarged elbow Reduced elbow flexion and extension ± Ulnar nerve palsy	
Rheumatoid arthritis	Autoimmune connective tissue disease Synovial joint inflammation Results in loss of joint space, joint erosions and joint destruction Often relapsing and remitting Typically middle-aged M:F ratio: ≈1:3 Rheumatoid factor positive in ≈70%	Gradual onset over ≥6 wks Fatigue Malaise Bilateral elbow pain and swelling Morning stiffness lasts ≥1 h	Fever Symmetrical joint involvement Enlarged elbows Tender swelling in acute synovitis ± Rheumatoid nodules ± Ulnar nerve palsy	Consider Sjogren's syndrome if dry eyes and dry mouth
Fractured olecranon	History of trauma or fall onto an outstretched hand	Pain and swelling of elbow ± Bruising ± Deformity	Bony tenderness ± Reduced elbow extension	
Dislocated elbow	History of fall onto outstretched hand with a flexed elbow	Pain and deformity of forearm Unable to extend elbow	Swollen elbow Elbow held in fixed flexion	Exclude an associated fracture

Foot pain

Diagnosis	Background	Key symptoms	Key signs	Additional information
Plantar fasciitis	Inflammation of the plantar fascia Age >40 yrs M<F Usually resolves within 6 wks	History of frequent activity (e.g. running) or Unaccustomed activity Pain felt on plantar surface of foot Worse on first few steps in the morning	Unilateral Antalgic gait Tenderness anterior to heel pad	
Gout	Disorder of purine metabolism Hyperuricaemia and urate crystal deposition Age 30–60 yrs M:F ratio: ≈20:1 Risk factors: Hyperuricaemia, high purine diet, excess alcohol, obesity, diuretics, hypertriglyceridaemia, family history	Acute onset symptoms Severe pain Malaise Erythema and swelling of joint Peaks within 24 h Painful movement of joint	Swollen joint Overlying erythema Warm on palpation ± Gouty tophi	*Commonly affected joints:* 1st MTP joint (Podagra) Knee Midtarsal joints Wrist Ankles Small hand joints Elbows
Morton's metatarsalgia (Morton's neuroma)	Entrapment of interdigital nerve between 3rd and 4th metatarsal heads Age 40–50 yrs M<F	Attacks of pain or paraesthesia on walking Radiates to toes	Tender in 3rd interdigital space Pain on squeezing forefoot	
Hallux valgus	Valgus deformity of 1st MTP joint M<F Risk factors: Tight footwear, high heels, gout, RA, hypermobility of joints, MS, Charcot-Marie-Tooth	Deformity of foot Pain in 1st MTP joint Inflamed bunion	Valgus deformity of 1st MTP joint Erythema of overlying skin Tenderness over bunion Reduced ROM of toe	Consider referral for surgical correction
Osteoarthritis of foot joints	Degenerative joint disease Risk factors: Advancing age, female gender, family history, previous joint injury, obesity	Pain in MTP and IP joints of feet Worse with activity Relieved by rest Joint stiffness lasts <30 mins in morning or after rest	Systemically well Antalgic gait Bony swelling and deformity Joint swelling and effusion Periarticular tenderness Pain on flexion or extension Reduced ROM of affected joints Crepitus	
Pes planus (Flat foot)	Medial arch normally develops after 2–3 yrs of walking	Nagging ache Worse on standing or walking	Medial border of foot almost touches the ground Arch not restored by standing on tiptoe	Only consider abnormal if associated with pain
Pes cavus (Arched foot)	Exaggerated mid-foot arch Usually idiopathic May occur secondary to neurological pathology (e.g. Charcot-Marie-Tooth, Friedreich's ataxia)	Pain under metatarsal heads or Pain over dorsum of toes	Bilateral High medial arch Heel in varus Clawing of toes Callosities over sole pressure points	Exclude neurological causes for deformity
Stress fracture	Commonly athletes, soldiers, dancers Often affects metatarsals, calcaneum and tibia	History of unaccustomed and repeated activity Pain initally after exercise Progresses to constant pain	Tender over fracture Warmth and swelling	
Talipes equinovarus (Club foot)	Fixed foot deformity Polygenic inheritance M:F ratio: ≈2:1	Foot is supinated and adducted Heel is higher than forefoot Abnormal gait	Unilateral or bilateral Talus and calcaneum point downwards (equinus) Navicular and forefoot rotated medially Foot cannot be passively everted and dorsiflexed ± Small heel and thin calf	Positional talipes is easily corrected with passive movement of foot. The foot can be dorsiflexed and everted until the toes touch the front of the leg
Rheumatoid arthritis (See Hand and wrist pain)				

Diagnosis	Background	Key symptoms	Key signs	Additional information
Acute osteomyelitis	Infection of bone marrow Via haematogenous (e.g. boil) or direct spread (e.g. minor abrasion) Results in inflammation, abscess formation and bone necrosis Commonly children or immunocompromised adults Risk factors: Trauma, DM, IVDU, chronic alcoholism, long-term steroid use, TB exposure, HIV/AIDS, sickle cell disease	Malaise Severe pain in affected limb ± History of injury or cellulitis ± History of septicaemia	Fever Acute tenderness in affected limb Localised pain Local erythema and swelling Localised warmth Reduced ROM of affected limb ± Discharging sinus tracts	Urgent admission for i.v. antibiotics Complications: Septic arthritis, bone deformity, chronic osteomyelitis, pathological fracture
Freiberg's disease	Osteochondritis of 2nd or 3rd metatarsal head Commonly teenagers and young adults M<F	Foot pain on walking Worse after unaccustomed activity	Antalgic gait Tender over affected metatarsal head	
Kohler's disease	Osteochondritis of navicular bone Age 2–10 yrs M>F	Pain over the dorsum of the midfoot	Antalgic gait Tender over the medial aspect of the foot	
Sever's disease	Osteochondritis of the calcaneum Age 10–13 yrs M>F	Gradual onset symptoms Heel pain Worse with activity Relieved by rest	Tender over calcaneum Pain on dorsiflexion of ankle Heel swelling	

Hand and wrist pain

Diagnosis	Background	Key symptoms	Key signs	Additional information
Fractured finger	History of hand trauma	Pain and swelling of finger Localised bruising	Finger deformity Tender over site of fracture	Refer to A&E for reduction
Carpal tunnel syndrome	Median nerve compression under the flexor retinaculum M<F Causes: Idiopathic, post-fracture, DM, hypothyroidism, menopause, pregnancy, dialysis, amyloidosis	Paraesthesia and pain Radiates to radial 3½ digits Worse at night Relieved by shaking wrist	Thenar muscle wasting Weakness of thumb apposition and grip *Positive Tinel's sign:* Tapping over carpal tunnel invokes paraesthesia *Positive Phalen's sign:* Wrist hyperflexion for ≥1 min invokes paraesthesia	
Work-related upper-limb pain (Repetitive strain injury)	Overuse syndrome	Pain in arm or wrist Worse with work-related activity	Normal upper limb examination	
Mallet finger	Avulsion of extensor tendon to the distal phalanx	History of injury to distal phalanx Typically caused by catching a fast hard ball Drooping of distal phalanx	Inability to actively straighten distal phalanx	
Gamekeeper's thumb (Skier's thumb)	Rupture of the ulnar collateral ligament	History of forced thumb abduction Very painful swollen thumb	Weak pincer grip	Refer for surgical repair
De Quervain's tenosynovitis	Inflammation of tendon sheath Age 30–50 yrs M<F	History of unaccustomed activity Pain over radial side of wrist Worse in the morning	Swelling over radial styloid Tenderness on palpation Pain induced on forced adduction and flexion of thumb	
Scaphoid fracture	History of fall onto outstretched hand	Pain over the wrist	Swelling over anatomical snuff box Tenderness on palpation	Risk of avascular necrosis of scaphoid X-rays may be normal for the first few weeks

Diagnosis	Background	Key symptoms	Key signs	Additional information
Osteoarthritis of the hand and wrist	Degenerative joint disease Results in loss of joint space, bone sclerosis, osteophyte formation Typically middle-age Risk factors: Advancing age, female gender, family history, previous joint injury, obesity	Pain and stiffness of fingers and wrist Worse with activity Relieved by rest Joint stiffness lasts <30 mins in morning or after rest Reduced hand function	Systemically well Hand muscle wasting Asymmetrical joint involvement Swollen MCP, PIP, DIP or wrist Heberden's nodes (DIP nodes) Bouchard's nodes (PIP nodes) Painful movement of affected joints Reduced ROM of fingers	
Rheumatoid arthritis	Autoimmune connective tissue disease Synovial joint inflammation Results in loss of joint space, erosions and joint destruction Often relapsing and remitting Typically middle-age M:F ratio: ≈1:3 Rheumatoid factor positive in ≈70%	Gradual onset over ≥6 wks Fatigue Malaise Weight loss Painful fingers, hands and wrist Morning stiffness lasts >1 h Soft tissue swelling of >3 joints Reduced hand function	Fever Hand muscle wasting Symmetrical joint involvement Swollen PIP, MCP or wrist Ulnar deviation of wrist Swan neck deformity Boutonniere deformity Rheumatoid nodules Painful movement of affected joints Reduced ROM of fingers and wrist *Systemic signs:* Sjorgren's syndrome Scleritis and episcleritis Leg ulcers Pericarditis Myocardial fibrosis Pulmonary fibrosis Polyneuropathy	*Other common joints affected:* MTP joints of the foot Ankles Knees Hips Cervical spine Shoulder
Raynaud's phenomenon	Digital ischaemia affecting peripheral arterioles			
Subtypes:				
Raynaud's disease	Onset teens to early 20s M<F Idiopathic Precipitated by cold or emotion	Intermittent attacks Worse in cold weather Fingers undergo colour change Pale (ischaemia) to blue (slow blood flow) to red (hyperaemia) Throbbing and aching fingers Finger swelling Attacks last minutes to hours	Bilateral Thumb often spared Systemically well Normal hand examination between atttacks Normal peripheral pulses No hepatosplenomegaly ± Digital ulceration ± Nail dystrophy	May also affect mouth, nose and toes
Raynaud's syndrome	Commonly associated with underlying disease Onset >30 yrs age Common causes: Systemic sclerosis SLE, RA, arteriosclerosis, migraine, DM, use of vibrating hand tools, smoking, previous frostbite, malignancy, lymphoma, drugs (e.g. beta-blockers)	Typically perennial symptoms Fingers undergo colour change Pale (ischaemia) to blue (slow blood flow) to red (hyperaemia) Throbbing and aching fingers Finger swelling Attacks last minutes to hours	Bilateral Systemically well Normal hand examination between attacks ± Digital ulceration	
Trigger finger	Nodule on middle or ring finger Becomes entrapped in tendon sheath Associated with: RA, DM, amyloidosis, dialysis	Finger remains in fixed flexion Can be flicked straight Mild pain on triggering finger	Palpable nodule at base of finger Nodule moves with tendon	
Behcet's disease (See Mouth ulcers)				
Keinbock's disease	Necrosis of lunate bone after injury Commonly young adults	Aching wrist Associated stiffness	Tender in centre and dorsum wrist Reduced wrist extension	

Hip pain

Diagnosis	Background	Key symptoms	Key signs	Additional information
Transient synovitis of hip (Irritable hip)	Usually occurs post-viral infection Age 2–12 yrs M:F ratio: ≈2:1 Usually resolves within 7–10 days	Limping child Pain in hip or knee ± Refusal to weight bear	Systemically well Hip held in slight flexion, abduction and external rotation Reduced ROM of hip Pain on hip extension and adduction	
Trochanteric bursitis	Associated with osteoarthritis May be triggered by repeated pressure over lateral hip	Pain over gluteal muscles and lateral thigh	Focal tenderness over greater trochanter Full ROM of hip	
Osteomalacia	Adult form of rickets Insufficent 1,25 dihydroxycholecalciferol (vitamin D3) Low calcium and phosphate Inadequate bone mineralisation Typical age >65 yrs Commonly South Asians Causes: Poor nutrition, lack of sun exposure, malabsorption, defective vitamin D metabolism in liver or kidney Stress fractures are common in: Femur, pubic rami, vertebra, ribs	Insidious onset symptoms Persistent fatigue Generalised bone pain and tenderness Often affects hip and lower back Difficulty rising from a chair ± Hypocalcaemia	Waddling gait Kyphosis or scoliosis Genu valgum Proximal muscle weakness	≈90% of vitamin D is obtained through sun exposure Children should be referred to a paediatrician
Osteoarthritis of the hip	Degenerative joint disease Major cause of hip pain Risk factors: Advancing age, family history, previous hip disease/trauma, obesity	Pain in groin, thigh or knee Worse with activity Relieved by rest (in early disease) Joint stiffness lasts <30 mins in morning or after rest	Systemically well Antalgic gait Muscle wasting around hip joint Painful movement Reduced internal rotation Reduced hip abduction ± Fixed flexion deformity (late stage)	
Hip fracture	Usually involves neck of femur Common in elderly M<F Risk factors: Falls, osteomalacia, osteoporosis	Often history of fall Pain and bruising around hip	External rotation and shortening of affected leg Reduced ROM of hip ± Able to weight bear	
Septic arthritis	Commonly affects knee or hip Can affect a prosthetic joint Often due to *Staphylococcus aureus* Commonly children <2 yrs age, elderly, immunosuppressed	Malaise Swollen joint Pain on active joint movement	Systemically unwell Fever Tachycardia Red hot swollen joint Affected limb held still Very painful on passive movement	Emergency admission for i.v. antibiotics
Malignancy (See Back pain)				
Rheumatoid arthritis (See Hand and wrist pain)				
Paget's disease of the bone	Abnormal osteoclast activity Disordered bone remodelling Results in larger and weaker bones Age >40 yrs M>F Commonly affects spine, skull and long bones ≈1% of cases develop sarcoma	Often asymptomatic or Dull bony pain Worse on weight bearing Progressive bone deformity Deafness	Bowing of tibia, femur and forearm Frontal bossing Deafness (CN VII compression) Osteoarthritis of adjacent joints Pathological fractures (e.g. femur)	

Diagnosis	Background	Key symptoms	Key signs	Additional information
Developmental dysplasia of the hip (**Congenital dislocation of the hip**)	Dysplastic or unstable hip joint Affects left hip > right hip M<F Risk factors: Family history, breech delivery, oligohydramnios, developmental abnormalities, first born	History of frequent falls Clicking hip ± Limping or waddling gait	Positive Ortolani and Barlow test in neonates *Positive Ortolani's sign:* Indicates hip dislocation Bilateral hip abduction reduces hip with a palpable clunk *Positive Barlow's sign:* Indicates a dislocatable hip Palpable clunk as hip dislocates backwards *Late signs:* Limping or waddling gait Asymmetrical leg creases Affected leg shorter Leg in external rotation Limited hip abduction Lumbar lordosis Increased perineal gap	Refer to orthopaedics for further investigation
Perthe's disease	Necrosis of the femoral head Age 3–11 yrs M:F ratio: ≈4:1 Heals over 2–3 yrs	Gradual onset symptoms ≥1 month Limping child Pain in hip or knee	Bilateral in ≈10% Initally all ROM painful Limited abduction and internal rotation of hip	Joint damage can lead to arthritis
Tuberculosis of bone	Reactivation of primary TB Ghon focus enlarges with lymphatic spread Commonly affects: Spine and large joints	Chronic symptoms Weight loss Malaise Joint pain and swelling Joint stiffness Plus respiratory symptoms (e.g. cough)	Usually involves one joint Muscle wasting Bone deformity Marked synovial thickening Full ROM is limited	
Slipped upper femoral epiphysis	Cartilaginous growth plate fracture Causes upper femoral epiphysis often to slip postero-inferiorly Commonly pubertal children M>F Associated with tall stature and obesity	Acute or gradual onset symptoms Pain at rest and on movement Pain in groin, anterior thigh or knee Limping gait ± History of hip trauma	Often unilateral Asymmetrical leg length Leg in external rotation Limited hip abduction and internal rotation	

Knee pain

Diagnosis	Background	Key symptoms	Key signs	Additional information
Bursitis	Prepatella or infrapatella subtypes possible	History of prolonged kneeling Anterior knee pain Knee swelling	Erythema and swelling over knee Tenderness on palpation Full ROM of knee	
Patella tendonitis	Inflammation of patella tendon Common in athletes	Insidious onset Anterior aching knee pain Pain occurs after or during activity	Tender over patella tendon Full ROM of knee	
Osteoarthritis of the knee	Degenerative joint disease Risk factors: Advancing age, female gender, family history, previous knee injury, obesity	Knee pain Worse with activity Relieved by rest Joint stiffness <30 mins in morning or after rest ± Pain on climbing stairs (Patellofemoral OA)	Systemically well Antalgic gait Bony swelling and deformity Quadriceps wasting Joint swelling and effusion Periarticular tenderness Crepitus Reduced ROM of knee Pain on knee flexion Joint instability	

Diagnosis	Background	Key symptoms	Key signs	Additional information
Meniscal tear	Commonly medial tears > lateral Often young adults	History of twisting injury to knee Severe pain Prevents further activity Worse with knee extended Swelling of knee over hours Locking of knee joint	Knee held in slight flexion Mild effusion Joint line tenderness McMurray's test: positive Apley's grind test: positive Apley's distraction test: negative	
Osgood-Schlatter's disease	Microfracture of tibial tubercle Caused by traction on patella tendon Commonly teenagers M>F Self-limiting within months	History of athletic acivity Anterior knee pain Onset of knee pain after activity	Swelling over tibial tubercle Tenderness on palpation Full ROM of knee	

Chondromalacia patellae	Softening of cartilage on articular
	  surface of patella
	Commonly teenagers
	M<F
		Anterior knee pain
		Worse on ascending and
		  descending stairs
			Tenderness on posterior surface
			  of patella
			Positive Clark's test:
			Pain on pressing patella against
			  femur with quadriceps
			  contracted	

Ilio-tibial band syndrome	Inflammation of ilio-tibial tract
	Commonly long-distance runners
	Age 15–50 yrs
		Non-specific pain over lateral side
		  of knee
		Worse on running, cycling,
		  climbing stairs
			Tenderness over lateral femoral
			  condyle or lateral tibial condyle
			Full ROM of knee	

Patellar dislocation	Lateral dislocation of patella
	Commonly teenagers
	M<F
		Spontaenous dislocation or
		History of direct blow to knee
		  with knee in slight flexion
		Painful knee
		Limited knee movement
			Knee held in flexion
			Patella visible on lateral side of
			  knee	

Gout (See Foot pain)				

Pseudogout	Calcium pyrophosphate
	  deposition
	Affects joint and periarticular
	  tissues
	Typically elderly
	Common risk factors:
	  Dehydration, illness,
	  hyperparathyroidism,
	  hypothyroidism, surgery/trauma
		Asymptomatic
		Or mimics mild gout
		Acute onset mild joint pain
		Erythema and swelling of single
		  joint
		Painful joint movement
		Commonly affected joints:
		  Shoulder, wrist, knee
			Joint effusion
			Overlying erythema
			Warm on palpation
			± Fever	

Psoriatic arthropathy	≈10% psoriasis patients affected
	Arthropathy occurs within 10 yrs
	  of disease onset
	Age 25–50 yrs
	Common joints affected:
	Knee
	Elbow
	DIP joints of fingers or toes
	Sacro-iliac joints
		Joint pain
		Joint stiffness
		Fatigue
		Malaise
		± Back pain
		± Photophobia
			Psoriatic plaques
			Asymmetrical or symmetrical joint
			  involvement
			Bony swelling and deformity
			Joint swelling and effusion
			Periarticular tenderness
			Crepitus
			Reduced ROM of affected joints
			Nail pitting
			± Sacro-ilitis
			± Sausage-shaped fingers
			± Achilles tendonitis
			± Iritis	

Medial collateral ligament injury	Most commonly injured knee
	  ligament
		History of valgus stress
		± Knee rotation
		Acute onset pain at time of injury
		Worsens over days
		Acute swelling post-trauma
			Knee held in slight flexion
			Swelling over medial side of knee
			Partial ligmament tear:
			Pain on stressing medial collateral
			  ligament
			Complete ligament tear:
			Painless opening of joint space
			Apley's grind test: negative
			Apley's distraction test: positive	

Diagnosis	Background	Key symptoms	Key signs	Additional information
Anterior cruciate ligament tear	Common causes: Sharp twisting knee injuries Valgus displacement and external knee rotation Blow to posterior tibia forces knee forwards in relation to femur Commonly athletes Age 14–30 yrs M<F	Acute onset pain "Popping sound" heard on injury Acute swelling and bruising post-trauma Giving way of knee	Painful swollen knee Periarticular bruising Reduced ROM of knee Positive Lachman test Positive anterior drawer test	
Septic arthritis	Commonly affects knee or hip Can affect a prosthetic joint Often due to *Staphylococcus aureus* Commonly children <2 yrs age, elderly, immunosuppressed	Malaise Swollen joint Pain on active joint movement	Systemically unwell Fever Tachycardia Red hot swollen joint Affected limb held still Very painful on passive movement	Emergency admission for i.v. antibiotics
Osteochondritis dissecans	Separation of bone fragment and articular surface from medial femoral condyle Separated fragment can become avascular or remain loose in joint Age 20–25 yrs M>F	History of trauma Intermittent knee ache or swelling Worse with activity Painful "clunk" on knee flexion or extension ± Knee locking or giving way (if loose body in knee)	External tibial rotation on walking Small knee effusion Full ROM of joint	Predisposes to OA of knee
Posterior cruciate ligament tear	Common causes: Knee forced backwards in relation to femur (e.g. dashboaord injury) Hyperextension of knee	Acute onset pain "Popping sound" heard on injury Acute knee swelling post-trauma Giving way of knee	Painful swollen knee Periarticular bruising Reduced ROM of knee Positive posterior drawer test	
Lateral collateral ligament injury	Usually associated with injury to posterolateral structures	History of direct blow to knee Acute onset pain Acute swelling post-trauma	Knee held in slight flexion Diffuse swelling *Partial ligmament tear:* Pain on stressing lateral collateral ligament *Complete ligament tear:* Painless opening of joint space Apley's grind test: negative Apley's distraction test: positive	
Hypermobility syndrome	General or local joint involvement Usually benign Commonly children or young adults Rarely associated with: Marfan's, Ehler-Danlos, Osteogenesis imperfecta	Recurrent joint pains Typically knee pain Worse after exertion	*Ligamentous laxity:* Elbow hyperextension Thumb hyperextension Hyperflexion of 5th MCP joint Knee hyperextension Palms can touch floor with knees extended	Severe laxity can increase risk of premature osteoartritis
Juvenile chronic arthritis (Still's disease)	Systemic inflammatory disorder Age <16 yrs M<F	Acute or gradual onset symptoms Fatigue Malaise Weight loss Joint pains Joint stiffness Myalgia ± Photophobia	Fever Antalgic gait Asymmetrical or symmetrical joint involvement Bony swelling and deformity Joint swelling and effusion Periarticular tenderness Crepitus Joint instability Reduced ROM of affected joints ± Salmon pink rash ± Uveitis ± Lymphadenopathy ± Hepatosplenomegaly	

Diagnosis	Background	Key symptoms	Key signs	Additional information
Rheumatic fever	Group A streptococcal infection Common in developing world Age 5–15 yrs Risk factors: Low socioeconomic status, overcrowded conditions	History of sore throat Onset symptoms 1–5 wks later Peristent fever Malaise Rash Painful swollen joints	Fever Migratory arthritis Lasts few hours to few days Inflamed swollen joints Periarticular tenderness Reduced ROM of affected joints ± Tachycardia ± Heart murmur ± Erythema marginatum ± Sydenham's chorea	Complications: Endocarditis and damage to heart valves

Muscle pain or weakness

Diagnosis	Background	Key symptoms	Key signs	Additional information
Muscle strain	Overuse injury Self-limiting	History of repetitive strain or unaccustomed activity Muscle pain hours after injury Worse on movement Relieved by rest	Systemically well Mild tenderness on palpation No arthralgia ± Swelling over affected muscle	
Cerebrovascular accident (See Dysphagia)				
Polymyalgia rheumatica	Inflammatory conditon Affects shoulder and pelvic girdle Age >50 yrs M:F ratio: ≈1:3	Pain around shoulders and pelvis Morning stiffness Difficulty getting out of bed Fatigue Weight loss Joint swelling	Fever Pain on active and passive movement of shoulders, neck, hips Muscle tenderness	Giant cell arteritis may co-exist
Medication	Common drugs: Fibrates, chloroquine, alcohol, corticosteroids, lithium, statins	Onset muscle weakness after taking medication ± Myalgia	Symmetrical involvement Proximal muscle atrophy Proximal muscle weakness Normal sensation	
Bells palsy	Lower motor neurone facial palsy Commonly age 15–45 yrs >80% recover spontaneously within 1–6 months	Acute onset within 24 h Unilateral facial drooping Unable to close eye Dribbling ± Recent history of post-auricular pain	Unilateral Unable to raise eyebrow Sagging mouth Unable to blow out cheeks On trying to close eye, eyeball rotates upwards and outwards (Bell's phenomenon) Reduced eye lacrimation Loss of taste ± Hyperacusis	Beware of corneal irritation and ulceration
Bornholm disease (See Chest pain)				
Fibromyalgia	Age 25–55 yrs M:F ratio: ≈1:7	Generalised body pain Insomnia Chronic fatigue Low mood Anxiety No arthralgia	Systemically well Depression Pain over specific trigger points No red flag signs	Red flag signs: Age <20 yrs or >55 yrs Abnormal neurology Thoracic pain Weight loss Fever History of malignancy Use of systemic steroids
Mononeuropathy	Entrapment of an individual peripheral or cranial nerve Associated with: DM, sarcoidosis, RA, polyarteritis nodosa, acromegaly, hypothyroidism, pregnancy	Numbness or paraesthesia Muscle weakness	Reduced sensation in distribution of affected nerve Reduced power in affected muscle group	

Diagnosis	Background	Key symptoms	Key signs	Additional information
Polymyositis	Autoimmune Inflammatory muscle condition Age 30–60 yrs May be associated with dermatomyositis and malignancy	Gradual onset over weeks/ months Progressive deterioration Fatigue Difficulty climbing stairs, rising from chair or combing hair Variable weakness ± Dysphagia	Symmetrical proximal muscle weakness Fine movements of hands impaired in late disease	
Charcot-Marie-Tooth syndrome (Peroneal muscular atrophy)	Autosomal dominant Progressive sensorimotor neuropathy Presents at puberty or early adulthood Peroneal muscles atrophy first then upper limbs	Gradual onset symptoms Progressive muscle weakness Muscle wasting Reduced sensation Difficulty with walking	Foot drop Pes cavus or pes planus Hammer toes Sensory loss in distal arms and legs Pain and temperature sensation usually intact Reduced power Absent reflexes throughout	
Myasthenia Gravis	Antibody-mediated autoimmune disorder ≈15% associated with thymoma ≈75% associated with thymic hyperplasia Precipitating factors include: Pregnancy, infection, drugs	Muscular fatigue Common muscles involved: Extra-ocular muscles, limbs, bulbar and or respiratory	Asymmetrical diplopia or ptosis Rapid muscle fatigue on exercise Shoulder girdle weakness > pelvic girdle weakness Normal tone, reflexes and sensation ± Facial weakness ± Dysarthria	Respiratory muscle involvement requires emergency airway management
Guillain-Barré syndrome	Neuromuscular paralytic syndrome Demyelination and axonal degeneration	Acute onset symptoms History of GI or URTI 1–3 wks ago Lower limb weakness Neuropathic pain in lower limbs Numbness in lower limbs Bladder dysfunction	Progressive symmetrical signs Ascending muscle weakness and sensory loss Facial muscle weakness Reduced sweating or heat tolerance Absent or reduced lower limb reflexes	Risk of respiratory muscle paralysis
Transverse myelitis	Acute inflammation Damages or destroys myelin Affects both sides of a segment of spinal cord Often due to viruses (e.g. Herpes, influenza, Epstein-Barr, varicella) Prognosis variable Recovery can take months to years	Onset over days or weeks Malaise Localised lower back pain or Shooting pains down legs Paraesthesia of legs Leg weakness Difficulty walking Allodynia (heightened sensation) Bowel and bladder dysfunction	Signs at and below affected level of spinal cord *LMN signs of lower limbs:* Muscle wasting Fasiculations Flaccid paralysis Absent or reduced reflexes Absent plantar response Sensory level in mid thoracic region	
Dystrophia myotonica	Autosomal dominant Most common muscular dystrophy Usual onset 15–40 yrs age Slowly progressive	Progressive muscle weakness	Muscle weakness Myotonia of face and limbs Symmetrical ptosis Normal pupils Absent limb reflexes ± Frontal baldness ± Cataract ± Infertility ± Mental impairment	
Duchenne muscular dystrophy	X-linked recessive Males age ≤3 yrs	Gradual onset symptoms Progressive muscle weakness Frequent falls Delayed walking	Inability to run and hop Waddling gait Pseudohypertrophic calf muscles Hypertonia of shoulders Proximal muscle weakness Gower's sign: positive	

Diagnosis	Background	Key symptoms	Key signs	Additional information

Poliomyelitis	Enterovirus affects CNS
	Faecal–oral or droplet spread
	Incubation ≈7–14 days
	More prevalent in developing
	  world
		Prodromal illness:
		Malaise
		Headache
		Sore throat
		Vomiting
		Diarrhoea
		± Muscle weakness 5–10 days
		  later
		Lower limbs > upper limbs
		Severe myalgia
			Fever
			LMN signs in affected muscles:
			Muscle wasting
			Fasiculations
			Flaccid paralysis of lower limbs
			Absent or reduced reflexes
			Absent plantar response
			Normal sensation
			± Diplopia
			± Dysphagia
			± Dysphonia
				Notifiable disease
				Risk of respiratory muscle
				  paralysis

Numbness and paraesthesia

Diagnosis	Background	Key symptoms	Key signs	Additional information

Panic disorder	History of discrete episodes of
	  anxiety (panic attacks)
	Intense subjective fear with
	  symptomatic manifestations
	Unanticipated attacks
	Variable in frequency
	Attack lasts <1 h
	Chronic anxiety >1 month
	Anxiety related to subsequent
	  attacks or effects of attack
	Agoraphobia may co-exist
	≈50% develop depression
		Fast palpitations
		Chest discomfort/pain
		Shortness of breath
		Dizziness
		Nausea/vomiting
		Numbness and tingling
		"Fear of losing control"
			No physical signs between
			  attacks
			During an attack:
			Hyperventilation
			Sweating
			Sinus tachycardia
			Hypertension
			Severe anxiety
			Affect congruent with mental
			  state
			Fear of death/illness
			± Suicidal ideation
				Exclude alcohol/drug misuse

Generalised anxiety disorder	Usually chronic persistent anxiety Excessive or unrealistic worry Inappropriate to the situation Affects daily functioning Associated with stress and depression	Fast palpitations Shortness of breath Dizziness Nausea/vomiting Numbness and tingling "Fear of losing control" Poor concentration Insomnia Urinary frequency Frequent or loose bowel motions Erectile dysfunction	Hyperventilation Sweating Sinus tachycardia Hypertension Severe anxiety Fear of death/illness Postural hand tremor	Exclude alcohol/drug misuse

Carpal tunnel syndrome	Median nerve compression under
	  the flexor retinaculum
	M<F
	Causes: Idiopathic, post-
	  fracture, DM, hypothyroidism,
	  menopause, pregnancy,
	  dialysis, amyloidosis
		Paraesthesia and pain
		Radiates to radial 3½ digits
		Worse at night
		Relieved by shaking wrist
			Thenar muscle wasting
			Weakness of thumb apposition
			  and grip
			Positive Tinel's sign:
			Tapping over carpel tunnel
			  invokes paraesthesia
			Positive Phalen's sign:
			Wrist hyperflexion for ≥1min
			  invokes paraesthesia	

Prolapsed lumbar disc	Prolapse of nucleus pulposus
	Impinges on lumbar nerve roots
	Age 20–50 yrs
	Associated with sciatica
		Low back pain
		Radiates to foot or toes
		Unilateral leg pain > low
		  back pain
			Paraesthesia in distribution of pain
			Straight leg raise induces pain
			Focal neurology limited to one
			  nerve root	

Migraine (See Headache)				

Diabetic neuropathy	Type I or Type II DM
	Sensory nerves affected > motor
	  nerves
	Risk factors: Chronic DM, poor
	  glycaemic control, smoking,
	  age >40 yrs, hypertension, IHD
		History of established diabetes or
		First presentation of undiagnosed
		  diabetes
		Commonly affects feet
		Numbness
		Paraesthesia
		Burning
		Symptoms worse at night
			Pes cavus
			Clawed toes
			Stocking distribution of reduced
			  sensation
			Absent ankle reflexes
			Injury or infection over foot
			  pressure points
			Painless ulceration
				Hands are also affected in severe
				  chronic disease

Diagnosis	Background	Key symptoms	Key signs	Additional information
Cerebrovascular accident (See Dysphagia)				
Cervical spondylosis	Chronic cervical disc degeneration Disc herniation, calcification and osteophytic outgrowths Age >40 yrs	Gradual onset symptoms Intermittent neck pain and stiffness Radiation to occiput, interscapular, upper limbs ± Paraesthesia of arm ± Weakness of arm	Usually unilateral Tender cervical spine Shoulder joint non-tender on palpation Reduced ROM of neck ± Sensory loss and hyporeflexia of upper limb	
Restless legs syndrome (Ekbom's syndrome)	Age >40 yrs M<F Risk factors: Iron deficiency, uraemia, pregnancy, DM, RA, polyneuropathy, family history	Uncomfortable feeling in arms and legs Temporary relief on movement of affected limbs Insomnia Depression Anxiety	Normal neurological examination	
Multiple sclerosis	Chronic condition Autoimmune demyelinating disorder Affects CNS only Commonly young adults M:F ratio: ≈2:3 Commonest cause of neurological disability in the young	Fatigue Blurred vision Visual loss Double vision Urgency Impotence Leg weakness Numbness or perineum and genitalia Bowel and/or bladder incontinence Paraesthesia of limbs Vertigo Incoordination	*Focal neurological deficit:* Symmetrical horizontal nystagmus Optic neuritis Cranial nerve lesions Cerebellar signs *UMN limb weakness:* No muscle wasting Spasticity Hypertonia Brisk reflexes Upgoing plantar response	
Mononeuropathy	Entrapment of an individual peripheral or cranial nerve Associated with: DM, sarcoidosis, RA, polyarteritis nodosa, acromegaly, hypothyroidism, pregnancy	Numbness or paraesthesia Muscle weakness	Reduced sensation in distribution of affected nerve Reduced power in affected muscle group	
Spinal stenosis	Narrowing of the spinal canal Due to hypertrophy at the posterior disc margin and facet joints Commonly >60 yrs age Causes: Chronic disc degeneration and OA	Aching of lower limbs Numbness and paraesthesia in lower limbs Symptoms worse on standing or walking for 10 mins Relieved by sitting or squatting against a wall to flex spine	*At rest:* Normal straight leg raise Normal lower limb pulses No focal neurology *Post-exertion:* Often unilateral signs Focal neurological signs in lower limbs	Unlike claudication, pain is not relieved by standing still
Polyarteritis nodosa	Necrotising vasculitis Aneurysms of medium arteries Ischaemia due to arterial thrombosis and stenosis Typically age 40–60 yrs M>F Multi-system disorder involving skin Lungs are often spared Associated with HBsAg	Malaise Weight loss Abdominal pain Testicular pain or tenderness Myalgia on exertion Raynaud's phenomenon	Fever Hypertension Episcleritis Livedo reticularis (net-like rash) TIA (e.g. unilateral blindness) Multiple mononeuropathy (sensory, motor or mixed) Heart failure Pericarditis *Abnormal urinalysis:* Haematuria Proteinuria	Urgent rheumatology referral If untreated, chronic renal failure is a common cause of death
Cauda equina syndrome	Common causes: Lumbar disc prolapse, spinal tumour or trauma, spinal abscess	Acute or gradual onset symptoms Low back pain Pain radiates to one or both legs Difficulty passing or stopping urine Faecal incontinence	Lower limb weakness Lower limb sensory deficit Absent lower limb reflexes Saddle anaesthesia ± Loss of anal tone and sensation	Refer for emergency admission Delayed treatment can cause permanent neurological deficit

Diagnosis	Background	Key symptoms	Key signs	Additional information
Lumbar cord compression	Common causes: Trauma, malignancy, prolapsed intervertebral disc *above* L1 level	Acute or gradual onset symptoms Paraesthesia in legs or perineum Difficulty passing or stopping urine Faecal incontinence	Tender lumbar vertebrae Lower limb weakness Lower limb sensory deficit Saddle anaesthesia *UMN signs in lower limbs:* Spasticity Hyperreflexia below level of lesion Upgoing plantars ± Loss of anal tone and sensation	Refer for emergency admission Delayed treatment can cause permanent neurological deficit
Compartment syndrome	Oedema in an osteofascial compartment Causes increased pressure and ischaemia of affected limb Risk factors: Limb injury, tight plaster cast	Painful limb Numbness Weakness Symptoms worse with activity	Pallor or cyanotic limb Swollen tissues Weak peripheral pulse Reduced sensation Reduced power in distal musculature Passive extension of fingers or toes increases pain	Presence of pulse does not exclude diagnosis

Shoulder pain

Diagnosis	Background	Key symptoms	Key signs	Additional information
Rotator cuff disorders	Commonest cause of shoulder pain			
Subtypes:				
Acute tendonitis	Age <40 yrs Pain subsides after a few days	History of repetitive shoulder use or heavy lifting Severe pain in upper arm Unable to lie on affected side	Painful active movement Painful but full passive movement ± Painful arc on abduction 60°–120°	
Subacromial impingement	Calcific rotator cuff tendon caught under coracoacromial arch Age 40–60 yrs	Pain on lifting arm Difficulty putting on a jacket Worse at night	Painful active movement Painful but full passive movement Painful arc on abduction 60°–120° Tender below anterior edge of acromion	
Rotator cuff tears	Age 45–75 yrs Risk factors: Shoulder trauma, chronic impingement (in elderly)	History of trauma or chronic impingment (leading to tear) Difficulty abducting arm	*Partial tears:* Painful active movement Painful but full passive movement *Large or complete tears:* Active abduction impossible from rest Active abduction possible from 90° Active lowering of arm from 90° causes sudden arm drop to side	
Adhesive capsulitis (Frozen shoulder)	Thickening and contraction of glenohumeral joint capsule with adhesion formation Results in progressive shoulder pain and stiffness Age 40–65 yrs M<F Risk factors: DM, thyroid disease Often resolves although full ROM may not return	Spontaneous onset or History of rotator cuff injury or immobility Unable to sleep on affected side 3 overlapping phases in history *Freezing phase:* Lasts 2–9 months Shoulder stiffness Pain on movement in all directions *Thawing/adhesive phase:* Lasts 4–12 months Shoulder stiffness Pain only at extremes of movement *Thawing/recovery phase:* Lasts 5–24 months Slow return of shoulder movement Full ROM may be incomplete	*Freezing phase:* Global limitation of shoulder movements Loss of external arm rotation and abduction by ≥50%	

Diagnosis	Background	Key symptoms	Key signs	Additional information
Cervical spondylosis	Chronic cervical disc degeneration Disc herniation, calcification and osteophytic outgrowths Age >40 yrs	Gradual onset symptoms Intermittent neck pain and stiffness Radiation to occiput, interscapular, upper limb ± Paraesthesia of arm ± Weakness of arm	Usually unilateral Tender cervical spine Shoulder joint non-tender or on palpation Reduced ROM of neck ± Sensory loss and hyporeflexia of upper limb	
Dressler's syndrome or MI (See Chest pain)				
Rheumatoid arthritis (See Hand and wrist pain)				
Cervical disc prolapse	Due to neck trauma or degenerative disease Symptoms are acute in trauma or gradual in degenerative disease C6 and C7 are most commonly affected Often resolves spontaneously	Neck stiffness Worse on coughing or straining Relieved by lying down Shooting pains radiate to occiput, interscapular, or upper limb Paraesthesia in distal limb	Usually unilateral Reduced ROM of neck Neck pain may be absent *Radiculopathy:* Upper limb wasting Proximal limb weakness Reduced sensation in C6 and C7 dermatomes Reduced or absent biceps and triceps reflex	
Osteoarthritis of the shoulder	Degenerative joint disease Shoulder commonly affected Age 50–60 yrs Risk factors: Congenital dysplasia, shoulder trauma	Shoulder pain Worse with activity Relieved by rest Shoulder stiffness	Systemically well Asymmetrical joint involvement Upper limb muscle wasting Restricted active and passive shoulder movements	
Polymyalgia rheumatica (See Muscle pain and weakness)				
Polymyositis (See Muscle pain and weakness)				

Swollen ankles

Diagnosis	Background	Key symptoms	Key signs	Additional information
Pregnancy	Increased fluid retention Uterine pressure on inferior vena cava Resolves post-partum	History of missed period or Positive pregnancy test Aching feet Gradual onset ankle and foot swelling Worst in hot weather and on standing Relieved by elevating legs	Bilateral pitting oedema Gravid uterus	
Medication	Common drugs: Calcium antagonists, NSAIDs, steroids	Onset of swelling after taking medication	Bilateral pitting oedema	
Cardiac failure (See Chronic breathlessness)				
Cellulitis	Infection of dermis and subcutaneous tissue Commonly streptococcal or staphylococcal infection	Pain over affected areas Spreading erythema and swelling Rapid progression ± Malaise	Often unilateral Well demarcated erythema Localised warmth and swelling ± Fever	Risk of skin necrosis if untreated Skin crepitus indicates anaerobic infection
Hypoalbuminaemia	Causes include: Liver disease, trauma, infection, malignancy, nephrotic syndrome, burns, haemorrhage, protein losing enteropathy, malnutrition	Symptoms vary depending on underlying cause	Bilateral pitting oedema Other signs according to underlying cause	

Diagnosis	Background	Key symptoms	Key signs	Additional information
Deep vein thrombosis	M<F Risk factors: Trauma or surgery, advancing age, obesity, smoking, long-haul flight, immobility, pregnancy, HRT, COCP, malignancy	Diffuse pain in calf Swelling of calf and ankle	Unilateral Low-grade fever <39°C Tachycardia Diffuse erythema Lower leg swelling Tender calf muscle *Positive Homan's sign:* Increased pain on dorsiflexion of foot	Consider PE if chest pain or SOB
Ruptured Baker's cyst	Synovial sac of knee joint herniates into popliteal fossa May rupture causing leakage of synovial fluid into calf Risk factor: Arthritic knee	Diffuse pain in calf Swelling of calf and ankle	Unilateral Diffuse erythema Swelling of lower leg Tender calf muscle *Positive Homan's sign:* Increased pain on dorsiflexion of foot	Mimics DVT which may co-exist
Compartment syndrome	Oedema in an osteofascial compartment Causes increased pressure and ischaemia of affected limb Risk factors: Limb injury, tight plaster cast	Painful limb Numbness Weakness Symptoms worse with activity	Pale or cyanotic limb Swollen limb Weak peripheral pulse Reduced sensation Reduced power in distal muscles Passive extension of fingers or toes increases pain	A palpable pulse does not exclude diagnosis
Pelvic tumour	Compression of inferior vena cava Results in lower limb oedema Causes include: Ovarian, renal, hepatic carcinoma	Gradual abdominal swelling Bloating Pelvic pain	Pelvic mass on abdominal and pelvic examination	
Post-thrombotic syndrome	Late complication of DVT	Gradual onset symptoms over years Chronic leg pain Chronic leg swelling	Typically unilateral "Beer bottle"–shaped lower leg Pitting oedema Varicose eczema Haemosiderin pigmentation Venous ulceration above medial malleolus	
Varicose veins	Incompetent valves cause blood flow from deep to superficial veins Risk factors: Venous hypertension from prolonged standing, pregnancy, pelvic tumour, previous DVT, family history Positive Trendelenburg test indicates sapheno-femoral incompetence	Prominent tortuous veins in legs Aching legs Pruritis	Pitting oedema Varicose eczema Venous ulceration Haemosiderin pigmentation ± *Positive Trendelenburg test:* Varicosity reducible on supine leg raise Controlled by groin pressure while standing Reappears after removing pressure	If trendelenburg test is negative, use a tourniquet further down the thigh and repeat test until level of incompetence is identified
Lymphoedema	Accumulation of fluid in subcutaneous tissues Can affect more than one limb M<F Common causes: Malignancy, post-surgery, trauma, pregnancy, infection, elephantiasis, yellow nail syndrome	Chronic symptoms Limb pain Limb swelling	Firm non-pitting oedema	Exclude pelvic tumour

Chapter 10
Skin, Hair and Nails

Blisters (bullae) or vesicles*

Diagnosis	Background	Key symptoms	Key signs	Additional information
Skin trauma	Subepidermal bullae Causes: Burns (cold, heat, chemical), friction, insect bites Self-limiting	Recent history of skin trauma Acute onset symptoms Painful bullae	Localised Tense bullae	
Oral herpes simplex virus (Cold sores)	Acute viral infection Typically due to HSV Type I			
Subtypes:				
Primary HSV	First episode of infection Common in pre-school children Spread by saliva Incubation 3–10 days Post-recovery, virus remains dormant in the sensory ganglia	Often asymptomatic or *Acute herpetic gingivostomatitis:* Painful mouth ulcers Bleeding gums	*Acute herpetic gingivostomatitis:* Fever Dehydration Cervical LN Ulceration of tongue, palate and buccal mucosa Multiple coalescing oral vesicles	
Recurrent HSV	HSV re-activation Trigger factors: Immunosupression, stress, sun exposure, menstruation Highly contagious Spread by saliva Spontaneous healing over 1–2 wks No scarring	Facial tingling and itching Followed by vesicle eruption within hours/days	Multiple weeping vesicles around mouth and nares Vesicles crust before healing	
Herpes zoster (Shingles) (See Chest pain and Painful eye)				
Varicella zoster (Chickenpox)	Commonly children age <10 yrs Incubation 1–3 wks Transmission: Airborne Infectivity begins a few days before rash Highly contagious More severe in adulthood Usually self-limiting Lifelong immunity is not absolute	Malaise Pruritis Affects: Face, neck and trunk	Fever Generalised rash Onset of rash over 3–5 days *Rash occurs at different stages:* Initially crops of macules Followed by papules then vesicles Vesicles dry and crust over ± Scarring (usually temporary)	Complications include encephalitis and pneumonia Erythema around lesions suggest secondary infection School exclusion for 6 days from onset of first rash Avoid contact with pregnant women, neonates and immunosuppressed. Seek medical advice if exposed

* Bulla: visible collection of fluid >5 mm; Vesicle: visible collection of fluid <5 mm.

Differential Diagnosis in Primary Care, 1st edition. By Nairah Rasul and Mehmood Syed. Published 2009 by Blackwell Publishing, ISBN: 978-1-4051-8036-8

Diagnosis	Background	Key symptoms	Key signs	Additional information
Impetigo	Superficial skin infection Highly contagious via skin contact Rapid spread			
Common subtypes:				

Bullous impetigo	*Staphyloccocus aureus* infection
	Commonly children age <2 yrs
	More prevalent in summer
	Risk factors: Eczema, allergic
	  dermatitis, grazed skin
	Scarring is uncommon
		Painless bullae
		Affects any part of the body
		Common area includes the face
			Large superficial bullae
			Clear or cloudy fluid-filled bullae
			Surrounding skin is erythematous
			  and itchy
			Bullae rupture
			Scab over with golden crust
			± Fever
				Consider admission in infants if
				  widespread infection

Non-bullous impetigo	Group A Streptococci and/or
	  Staphyloccocus aureus infection
	Commonly school-aged children
	More prevalent in summer
	Risk factors: Eczema, allergic
	  dermatitis, grazed skin
	Scarring is uncommon
		Painless itchy pustules
		Affects any part of the body
		Common area includes the face
			Tiny superficial pustules or vesicles
			Surrounding skin is erythematous
			Lesions rupture easily
			Scab over with golden crust
			Moist and erythematous skin
			Regional LN
				School exclusion until lesions have
				  crusted and healed
				In severe and recurrent
				  staphylococcal infection,
				  consider DM

Hand, foot and mouth disease	Caused by Coxsackie enterovirus
	Commonly <5 yrs age
	Spread by faecal–oral route
	Self-limiting within 1 wk
		Malaise
		Anorexia
		Followed by mouth ulcers and
		  then skin lesions
		± Pruritis
			Mild fever
			Mouth lesions:
			Multiple yellow ulcers
			Surrounded by erythematous halo
			Hand and foot lesions:
			Erythematous macules form grey
			  vesicles on erythematous base
			Skin rash:
			Erythematous maculopapular rash
				NOT related to cattle "Foot and
				  mouth" disease

Pompholyx	Eczema affecting palms and soles
	Acute or recurrent condition
	Typical age 20–40 yrs
	M:F ratio: ≈1:2
	Risk factors: Perspiration, allergic
	  dermatitis, emotional stress
	Vesicles usually resolve
	  spontaneously within 4 wks
		Acute onset symptoms
		Itching or burning of palms/soles
		Followed by vesicle eruption
			Transluscent itchy vesicles
			Affects palms and soles
			Vesicles may rupture
			Erythematous scaling skin
			Sweaty palms and soles
				Secondary infection is common

Erythema multiforme
 	
	Age <40 yrs
	Trigger factors include: HSV,
	  hepatitis, *Streptococcus*,
	  radiotherapy
	Often mild
	Usually self-limiting within 3 wks
		Acute onset symptoms
		Non tender skin rash
		Affects: Mouth, genitals, palms,
		  soles, extensor surfaces of arms
		  and legs
			Target lesions:
			Round macular erythematous
			  lesions
			Purplish centre with pale outer ring
			Symmetrical peripheral
			  distribution
			Spreads centrally
			± Blistering of lesions
				Stevens-Johnsons syndrome:
				A severe drug-induced form
				  involving the mucous
				  membranes

Oedema blisters	Due to rapid onset severe oedema
	Commonly affects lower limb
	Causes of oedema:
	  CCF, immobility, DVT,
	  hypoproteinaemia, lymphatic
	  obstruction
		Painless bullae	Superficial tense bullae
			Limited to areas of oedema
			± Serous exudate
				Bullae resolve with the oedema

Fixed drug reaction	Skin reaction occurs in same site(s)
	  each time offending drug is taken
	Common drugs: Sulphonamides,
	  tetracyclines, barbiturates,
	  laxatives containing
	  phenolphthalein
	Re-exposue reactivates old and
	  new lesions
	Hyperpigmentation can last
	  months
		Onset rash after taking drug
		May occur ≤2 wks post-ingestion
		Commonly affects: Lips, limbs,
		  genitalia
		± Pain or burning
		± Pruritis
			Single or multiple lesions
			Well demarcated
			Round/oval patch or plaque
			Erythematous with purplish centre
			± Central bulla or necrosis
			Rash lasts days to weeks
			Fades slowly
			Residual post-inflammatory
			  hyperpigmentation	

Diagnosis	Background	Key symptoms	Key signs	Additional information
Dermatitis herpetiformis	Chronic autoimmune condition Granular IgA deposits in dermal papillae Age 20–30 yrs Associated with gluten-sensitive enteropathy (coeliac disease) GI symptoms often absent	Intensely itchy and burning rash Affects: Scalp, shoulders, elbows, buttocks, knees, shins	Symmetrical Groups of tiny erythematous papules and vesicles Excoriated skin and vesicles Oral mucosa not affected	
Bullous pemphigoid	Autoimmune disorder Commonly age >70 yrs Rarely affects mucous membranes Subepidermal bullae Antibodies to Type XVII collagen of the dermo-epidermal junction Often self-limiting after >5 yrs	Typically an initial pruritic rash Followed by skin blistering Commonly affects: Limbs, armpits, groins ± Mouth in ≈20%	Large tense blood-stained bullae On erythematous urticarial base Do not rupture easily Blisters rupture or are reabsorbed Form crusts Rapid healing without scarring	Cicatricial pemphigoid affects mucous membranes only and is associated with scarring
Pemphigus	Group of autoimmune disorders ≈70% are Pemphigus vulgaris Commonly 30–70 yrs age Most prevalent in Asians and Ashkenazi Jews Affects skin and mucosal surfaces Epidermal bullae IgG autoantibodies often present in skin and serum Associated with myasthenia gravis	Painful skin blistering Not itchy Commonly affects: Mouth, perineum, genitals	*Skin lesions:* Flaccid superficial bullae On normal or erythematous base Painful bullae Rupture easily Slow-healing weepy erosions Peri-lesional skin slides away easily (Nikolsky's sign) *Oral lesions:* Flaccid superficial bullae or erosions Irregular and poorly defined Painful Affects: Gums, buccal mucosa, palate Slow-healing erosions	Secondary infection is common Eating and drinking may be difficult
Eczema herpeticum	HSV infection Type I or II Affects pre-existing eczema Causes widespread infection	Acute onset symptoms Areas of rapidly worsening eczema Painful rash Commonly affects face and neck ± Rapid spread to other parts	Clusters of small bullae Filled with yellow pus Punched out shallow circular ulcers Size 1–3 mm in diameter May coalesce ± Fever ± Lymphadenopathy	Consider hospital admission if systemically unwell
Epidermolysis bullosa	Inherited condition Severity determined by type Skin and mucous membrane blistering on minimal trauma Associated with GORD	Blistering of limbs, extremities and mucus membranes Follows minimal skin friction/ trauma	Clusters of bullae Hyperkeratosis of skin	
Porphyria cutanea tarda	Commonest type of porphyria Uroporphyrinogen decarboxylase deficiency Involved in hepatic haem synthesis Age >40 yrs Autosomal dominant or sporadic after exposure to certain drugs Common drugs: Oestrogen, alcohol, iron, chlorinated phenols	Skin blistering Affects sun-exposed skin Common areas: Dorsum hands, face, forearms Pruritis	Erosions and small bullae Fragile sun-exposed skin Skin heals with scarring and hyperpigmentation Facial hypertrichosis	Sporadic PCT is associated with hepatitis C, haemochromatosis and HIV

Facial Erythema

Diagnosis	Background	Key symptoms	Key signs	Additional information
Acne vulgaris	Chronic inflammatory condition Due to: Increased sebum, blocked hair follicles, *Propionibacterium acnes* colonisation, inflammation Not diet-related Typically affects adolescents	Greasy skin and hair Recurrent red spots Affects: Face, nape, shoulders, back, chest	*Closed comedones (whiteheads):* Pearly papules *Open comedones (blackheads):* Dilated blocked hair follicles *Inflammatory lesions:* Erythematous papules or pustules Itchy and/or painful Resolve and recur over days Tender nodules and cysts ± Deep "ice-pick" scars	
Acne rosacea	Chronic inflammatory condition Commonly middle-aged women Prevalent in Celtic skin type Trigger factors: Topical steroids, stress, alcohol, hot drinks, UV light ≈50% have eye problems	Intermittent facial flushing ± Eye symptoms (e.g. grittiness)	Crops of papules and/or pustules Fixed erythema Telangiectasia Thickening of skin Affects: Forehead, cheeks, nose tip, chin No comedones No scaling ± Eye problems (e.g. blepharitis, conjunctivitis)	In men, severe involvement of the nose causes Rhinophyma
Facial seborrhoeic dermatitis	Inflammatory reaction to *Malassezia furfur* yeast A normal skin commensal Typical onset at puberty Affects sebum-rich areas (e.g. face, presternal area, upperback, flexures) High recurrence Severe in AIDS	Itchy scaly face and scalp Persistent dandruff Worse with stress, fatigue, ill health ± Scalp hair loss	Erythema and white/yellow thick scales Affects: Hairline, forehead, ears, nasolabial folds, eyebrows Severe dandruff ± Blepharitis ± Otitis externa	
Scarlet fever	Group A beta-haemolytic Streptococci Produces erythrogenic toxin Nasopharynx carriage in 10%–15% of healthy persons Commonly children age 4–8 yrs Droplet spread Incubation ≈2 to 4 days Often associated with pharyngitis ≈10% streptococcal throat infections evolve into scarlet fever	Sore throat Headache Abdominal pain Malaise Myalgia Rash	Fever Facial flushing Circumoral pallor *Onset of rash 12–48 h post-fever:* Pinpoint dark red papules on erythematous base Marked in skinfolds Blanches on pressure Spreads from head to toe ± Desquamation post-rash Enlarged oedematous tonsils Tender cervical LN Initially white furred tongue Becomes "strawberry red" (red papillae) ± White tonsillar exudate ± Haemorrhagic spots on palate	School exclusion 5 days from starting antibiotics

Diagnosis	Background	Key symptoms	Key signs	Additional information
Erysipelas	Due to beta-haemolytic Streptococcus skin innoculation Peak age 60–80 yrs Risk factors: Inflammatory dermatoses, skin trauma, nasopharyngeal infection, dermatophyte infections, poor hygiene, DM, alcohol abuse, immunodeficient, nephrotic syndrome	Prodromal malaise and chills Followed by sudden onset symptoms Pruritis Burning sensation Tender skin Red skin patch Enlarges over 3–6 days Affects face or legs Anorexia Fatigue Arthralgia	High-grade fever >39°C Shiny plaque Deep erythema Sharply demarcated Raised edges Skin oedema Indurated Warm and tender skin ± Vesicles and bullae	Compared with cellulitis, erysipelas is more sharply demarcated and has raised edges
Rubella (German measles)	Mild RNA viral illness Incubation 2–3 wks Droplet spread Usually self-limiting within 10 days	Prodromal malaise (common in adults) Headache Pink rash Affects: Face then trunk then limbs Lasts up to 4 days Gritty eyes ± Arthralgia	Fever Conjunctivitis Pink discrete macules that coalesce No skin desquamation or scarring Cervical LN Post-auricular and sub-occipital LN ± Petechiae on soft palate	Notifiable disease School exclusion for 5 days post onset rash Associated with teratogenicity in first trimester pregnancy
Erythema infectiosum (Fifth disease)	Human parvovirus B19 infection Winter and spring epidemics Occur every 4–7 yrs Commonly nursery and school-aged children Droplet and parenteral spread Incubation 4–20 days Only infectious prior to onset rash Usually self-limiting	Coryzal symptoms Headache Sore throat ± Symmetrical arthralgia	Mild fever Cervical LN Maculopapular erythematous facial rash Resembles "slapped cheek" Spreads to arms and legs Fades to a lacy rash Rash lasts up to 1 wk	Can cause miscarriage and Hydrops fetalis in pregnancy
Systemic lupus erythematosus	Multisystem autoimmune disease Affects skin and internal organs Relapsing and remitting episodes Severity varies Age 30–40 yrs M:F ratio: ≈1:9 Prevalent in SE Asians and Afro-Carribeans Associated with: anti-dsDNA, low complement C3/C4, ANA: Ro, La, Sm, RNP ≈20%–35% have antiphospholipid syndrome Drug-induced SLE uncommon	*Skin symptoms:* Painful mouth or nasal ulcers Hair loss Skin photosensitivity *Systemic symptoms:* Fatigue Malaise Weight loss Arthralgia (e.g. hands) Myalgia Shortness of breath Pleuritic chest pain Low mood	*Skin signs:* Facial erythema ("butterfly" rash) Worse with sun exposure Diffuse alopecia Maculopapular rashes Mucosal ulceration Livedo reticularis Raynaud's phenomenon *Systemic signs:* Fever Anaemia Hypertension Lymphadenopathy Peripheral symmetrical flitting arthritis (non-erosive) Pleural effusion Lung crepitations (Fibrosing alveolitis) Pericardial rub (pericarditis) Psychosis and/or seizures Splenomegaly	Complications include: Glomerulonephritis, stroke, CHD Clinical signs may appear simultaneously or serially
Dermatomyositis	Autoimmune disease Affects skin and skeletal muscles Adults age 45–65 yrs or children Children have more non-muscular problems (e.g. GI ulcers and infections) Adults >60 yrs age often have malignancy	Malaise Weight loss Myalgia Muscle weakness Arthralgia Rash ± Dysphagia (pharyngeal weakness)	Fever Heliotrope rash (red–mauve discolouration of eyelids) Erythematous macular rash Affects face and upper trunk Violaceous scaly rash on knuckles Thickened finger cuticles Nailfold telangiectasia Profound proximal symmetrical muscle weakness Insignificant muscle wasting Normal sensation and reflexes	

Diagnosis	Background	Key symptoms	Key signs	Additional information
Mitral stenosis (See Heart murmurs)				

Toxic erythema
(Erythema toxicum
neonatorum)
	Benign self-limiting skin eruption
	Predilection for hair-bearing areas
	Commonly full-term newborns
	Onset within first 4 days of life
	Not inherited or infectious
	Spontaneously resolves within
	  2 wks
	No sequelea
	Rarely recurs
		No lethargy
		No irritability
			No fever
			Well child
			Maculopapular erythematous rash
			Irregular brown–red macules
			Vary in size and number
			Rash blanches
			Affects: Face, trunk, proximal
			  limbs
			Palms and soles rarely affected
				Exclude history of maternal
				  infection

Hair loss

Diagnosis	Background	Key symptoms	Key signs	Additional information
Androgenic alopecia **(Common balding)**	Occurs with advancing age Due to androgens Commonly age >30 yrs M>F			
Subtypes:				
Male-pattern balding		Gradual hair loss Commonly from temples and crown	Circumscribed hair loss Normal scalp	

Female-pattern hair loss	Often less severe and slower
	  progression
	Typically Ludwig-pattern hair loss
		Gradual onset hair loss/thinning	*Ludwig-pattern hair loss:*
			Normal scalp
			Front hair line preserved
			Thinning/hair loss at centre parting
			or
			Hamilton-pattern hair loss:
			Male-pattern balding
			Hair loss from temples and crown
			No menstrual disturbance
			± Mild hirsutism
				Consider androgen-secreting
				  tumour if severe hirsutism or
				  virilisation

Alopecia areata	Probably autoimmune
	Childhood or young adults
	Spontaneous hair growth usually
	  occurs over months
	Hair may regrow white initially
	High recurrence over 5 yrs
	Hair loss can be permanent
	Associated with thyroid disease
	  and vitiligo
		Rapid onset hair shedding
		Affects any hair-bearing part (e.g.
		  scalp, eyebrows, beard)
		± Spread to entire scalp (totalis)
		  or body (universalis)
			Normal scalp
			Round or oval patch of hair loss
			Often singular but can be
			  mutliple
			Patches may coalesce
			  "Exclamation mark hairs" at
			  margins of depleted areas
			± Nail changes (pitting, Beau
			  changes)	

Contact allergic dermatitis	Inflammation post-exposure to a
	  particular chemical(s)
				Consider occupation and ask
				  about hobbies

Subtypes:				

Allergic dermatitis	Affects certain people
	Prior sensitisation to an allergen
	Reaction delayed >24 h
	Common allergens: Nickel,
	  cosmetic preservatives,
	  perfumes
		Delayed onset symptoms
		Itchy sore skin
		Thinnest skin areas often affected
		  first (e.g. around eyes, back
		  of hands)
			Acute exposure:
			Skin inflammation and erythema
			Weeping vesicles
			± Spread to nearby sites not in
			  direct contact
			Chronic exposure:
			Dry scaly fissured skin	

Irritant dermatitis	Can affect anyone
	No prior sensitisation
	Direct contact damages skin
	Rapid reaction 6–12 h post first
	  exposure
	Common allergens: Dyes, acid/
	  alkalis, soap, detergent,
	  persistent moisture
		Acute onset symptoms
		Worse with repeated exposure
		Itchy sore skin
			Acute exposure:
			Skin inflammation and erythema
			Weeping vesicles
			Rash often localised
			Chronic exposure:
			Dry scaly fissured skin	

Diagnosis	Background	Key symptoms	Key signs	Additional information
Tinea capitis (Scalp ringworm)	Dermatophyte fungal infection Invades hair shaft Common types in UK: *Trichophyton tonsurans* (anthropophilic) *Microsporum canis* (zoophilic) Typically pre-pubertal children High prevalence in urban communities Transmission via: Contact with infected persons, cats/dogs, or airborne	Itchy scalp	≥1 patch(es) of partial hair loss Scaly scalp Broken hairs above or at scalp level ± Kerion (boggy tender scalp and pustules with cervical LN)	Carriers may have no clinical signs or symptoms Nail and skin can become infected Complications include scarring alopecia and permanent hair loss
Traction alopecia	Due to chronic tight hairstyles Commonly girls, Sikh boys, Afro-Carribeans	Gradual hair loss	Normal scalp Hair thinning/loss around scalp margin	
Seborrhoeic dermatitis (See Facial erythema)				
Telogen effluvium	Hair growth enters telogen phase Growth ceases and hair falls out 6–10 wks later Occurs ≈3 months post major stress Causes of major stress include: Illness, surgery, childbirth, anorexia/bulimia Often resolves spontaneously within a few months	History of recent stressful event General hair loss and thinning Noticeable on washing hair	Normal scalp No bald patches Generalised thinning of hair Hair is pulled out easily	If hair loss persistent, consider iron deficiency and hypothyroidism
Systemic lupus erythematosus (See Facial erythema)				
Drug-induced hair loss	Common drugs: Cytotoxic drugs, anti-thyroids, anticoagulants, vitamin A analogues Hair loss is temporary	Onset hair loss after taking medication	Normal scalp Generalised hair loss	
Morphoea (See Scales and Plaques)				
Trichotillomania	Compulsive hair pulling, usually involves the scalp Associated with anxiety, OCD, depression, family conflict	Low self-esteem Habitual hair pulling Worse with stress	Normal scalp Patches of localised hair loss	May affect any area of hair growth

Hirsutism

Diagnosis	Background	Key symptoms	Key signs	Additional information
Physiological	Excessive hair growth in females Male distribution of terminal hair Familial in South Asians, Mediterraneans Associated with obesity and advancing age	Slow onset post-puberty Excessive thick dark hair Affects: Face, lower abdomen, innner thighs, back, chest No oligo/amenorrhoea	Mild hirsutism Systemically well No virilisation	
Anorexia nervosa (See Amenorrhoea/ Oligomenorrhoea)				
Polycystic ovarian syndrome	Pre-menopausal women Associated with insulin resistance and infertility ≥2 of the following: Symptomatic Elevated LH (or FSH during menses) and supressed SHBG Polycystic ovaries on ultrasound	Asymptomatic or Irregular or absent menses Excess body hair Frontal balding	± BMI >30 kg/m² ± Acne ± Hirsutism	Weight loss is beneficial

Diagnosis	Background	Key symptoms	Key signs	Additional information
Medication	Common drugs: Anabolic steroids, danazol, minoxidil, metoclopramide, methyldopa, phenothiazines, progestogens	Onset of hair growth after taking medication	Mild hirsutism	
Late-onset congenital adrenal hyperplasia	Autosomal recessive Usually 21-hydroxylase deficiency Results in cortisol deficiency and androgen excess Onset late childhood or early adulthood Associated with female infertility and PCOS	May be asymptomatic or Oligo- or amenorrhoea Excess hair growth	Precocious puberty Onset ≈8 yrs age in both sexes Acne ± Virilisation ± Hirsutism	
Cushing's syndrome	Causes: Cushing's disease, iatrogenic glucocorticoid excess, adrenal tumour, small cell lung carcinoma Commonly 30–50 yrs age M<F Associated with osteoporosis	Increase in abdominal girth Irregular menses or amenorrhoea Excess body hair Easy bruising Impotence	Hypertension Moon face Acne Interscapular fat pad (buffalo hump) Purple/red abdominal striae Truncal obesity Thin pigmented skin Hirsutism Proximal muscle weakness	
Adrenocortical carcinoma	An aggressive tumour Typically children or young adults Presentation depends on which adrenal hormone(s) is excessive: Glucocorticoid–Cushing's syndrome Androgen–Virilisation Aldosterone–Conn's syndrome Oestrogen–Feminisation Associated with MEN 1 and 2	Vary depending on underlying hormone syndrome ± *Cushing's syndrome* ± *Virilisation in females:* Amenorrhoea Excess body hair Deep voice ± *Conn's syndrome:* Palpitations ± *Feminisation in males:* Loss of libido Impotence	Vary depending on underlying hormone syndrome ± *Cushing's syndrome* ± *Virilisation in females:* Male-pattern balding Acne Hirsutism Truncal obesity Increase shoulder muscle mass Clitoris hypertrophy ± *Conn's syndrome:* Confusion Hypertension Muscle weakness (hypokalaemia) ± *Feminisation in males:* Gynaecomastia	Urgent referral
Ovarian carcinoma (See Lower abdominal mass)				

Hyperpigmentation

Diagnosis	Background	Key symptoms	Key signs	Additional information
Chloasma	Increased melanin M:F ratio: ≈1:9 Can occur spontaneously Risk factors: Asian/Hispanic skin, pregnancy, COCP, sun exposure, family history	Gradual darkening of skin Worse after sun exposure	Macular symmetrical rash Tan to brown/black hyperpigmentation Affects sun-exposed areas: Forehead, cheeks, chin	
Post-inflammatory hyperpigmentation	Melanosis of epidermal or dermal layer Typically affects pigmented skin: Indian, African Causes: Inflammatory dermatoses (e.g. acne), trauma, UV exposure, drugs (e.g. chlorpromazine), allergy, chemicals (e.g. silver, arsenic) Resolution may take years	History of recent skin disorder (e.g. inflammation, itching, scaling) Followed by gradual darkening of skin	Brown macular rash Irregular border	

Diagnosis	Background	Key symptoms	Key signs	Additional information
Pityriasis versicolor (see Hypopigmentation)				
Chronic renal failure (See Gynaecomastia)				
Acanthosis nigricans	Papillomatous hyperpigmentation of epidermis Usually benign in young adults Associated with insulin resistance Typically affects obese adults Commonly darker skin races Associated with GI adenocarcinoma in older patients	Darkening and thickening of skin ± Pruritis	Discrete symmetrical rash Brown–black hyperpigmentation Velvety appearance Initially macular Progresses to palpable plaques Affects: Axillae, goin, posterior neck ± Skin tags	Weight reduction may result in resolution
Neurofibromatosis Type 1 (Von Recklinghausen's disease)	Neurocutaneous disorder Autosomal dominant Affects chromosome 17 Spontaneous mutation occurs in ≈50% Café-au lait macules may be present at birth Malignant sarcomatous change occurs in ≈15% of neurofibromas	Increase in size and number of café-au lait macules during first 10 yrs Onset neurofibromas post-adolescence	>6 Café-au-lait macules 0.5 to 5 cm in diameter Affect trunk and limbs Brown axillary or inguinal freckles (pathognomonic) Up to 0.3 cm in diameter *Dermal neurofibromas:* Skin-to-tan coloured nodules Soft or rubbery on palpation Random or localised ± Pedunculated *Subcutaneous neurofibromas:* Less well circumscribed Deeper and firmer on palpation ± *Plexiform neurofibromas (≈10%):* Tender nodules along a nerve Commonly cervical or trigeminal	Non-cutaneous features inlcude: Congenital glaucoma, seizures, kyphoscoliosis, short stature, tibial bowing, precocious puberty, learning difficulties, hypertension
Peutz-Jegher's syndrome	Autosomal dominant Associated with multiple GI hamartomatous polyps Increased risk: GI carcinoma, intussusception, intestinal bleeding	History of abdominal pain History of childhood intussusception	Brown macules (lentigines) Affects: Buccal mucosa, lips, palms, soles, anogenital May fade after puberty	High risk of malignancy: GI, breast, lung, ovary and pancreas Warrants regular endoscopy surveillance
Addison's disease	Primary adrenal insufficiency Commonest cause: Autoimmune Precipitated by: Trauma, stress, infection, infarction Autoimmune diseases often co-exist (e.g. IDDM, Graves' disease)	Insidious onset symptoms Lethargy Weakness Anorexia Weight loss Nausea/vomiting Diarrhoea ± Severe abdominal pain	Vitiligo Postural hypotension *Hyperpigmentation of:* Palmar creases Buccal mucosa Axillae Scars	Abrupt withdrawal/reduction in chronic steroids can provoke an Addisonian crisis Shock and hypoglycaemia warrant an emergency admission
Classical Haemachromatosis (See Jaundice)				

Hypopigmentation

Diagnosis	Background	Key symptoms	Key signs	Additional information
Vitiligo	Skin depigmentation Loss of melanocytic activity Probably autoimmune Commonly age 10–30 yrs Localised or generalised Vitiligo patches do not tan Risk factors: Family history, thyroid antibodies, pernicious anaemia, DM, Addison's disease, chemical skin exposure, repeated skin trauma Repigmentation may occur spontaneously in children	Gradual onset symptoms Asymptomatic patches of skin depigmentation Patches increase in size and number Become confluent Common areas: Perioral, periocular, hands, scalp ± White or grey scalp hair	Depigmented macules Clearly circumscribed Usually symmetrical Variable and irregular in size and shape	
Pityriasis alba	Mild eczema Typically children age 3–16 yrs Commonly darker skin races Usually resolves within a few years	Erythematous patches Resolve and become pale Usually asymptomatic Affects: Face, upper arms, trunk	Multiple lesions Pale hypopigmented macules Fine scaly surface Variable size and shape	
Pityriasis versicolor	*Overgrowth of Malassezia* yeast A normal skin commensal Present in pilosebaceous follicles Commonly adolescents Affects all skin types Risk factors: Humid climate, hyperhidrosis Not infectious High recurrence	Large irregular skin patches Affects trunk and arms Rarely affects face ± Mild pruritis	*Hyperpigmentation in fair skin:* Pink or light brown macular rash Fine scaly surface *Hypopigmentation in dark skin:* Patchy hypopigmented macules Fine scaly surface	Hypopigmented patches may take several months to resolve
Post-inflammatory hypopigmentation	Destruction of melanocytes Common causes: Eczema, psoriasis, burns, scars, cryotherapy	History of skin disorder or trauma	Patches of hypopigmentation Usually localised	
Sutton's halo naevus	An immune response to a melanocytic naevus Benign Onset around puberty Usually resloves spontaneously over years	Asymptomatic brown naevus Commonly affects trunk No irritation, bleeding, ulceration	Single or multiple naevi Central uniformly pigmented naevus Round or oval in shape Followed by depigmentation of uniform width around the naevus ± Naevus involution ± Subsequent naevus repigmentation over years	

Diagnosis	Background	Key symptoms	Key signs	Additional information
Lichen sclerosis et atrophicus	Chronic inflammatory dermatosis Affects urinary and sexual function Commonly middle-aged women and prepubertal girls M:F ratio: ~1:7 Associated with balanitis xerotica obliterans Prepubertal lesions usually resolve by menarche	Itchy and sore rash Dysuria Superficial dyspareunia Pain on defaecation Affects genitals in both sexes (vulva, perineum, perianal, foreskin, glans) ± Extra-genital areas in ≈20% (e.g. scars or areas of repeated trauma)	Initially erythematous patches Become white atrophic plaques Shiny surface ± Blistering and purpura	Complications include vaginal stenosis or phimosis Genital lesions are at risk of squamous cell carcinoma
Tuberous sclerosis	Autosomal dominant or sporadic Multisystem disorder Hamartomatous malformation (benign tumour) of skin and internal organs Common organs affected: Skin, eyes, brain, kidneys, heart Associated with autistic spectrum disorder	Typical onset in infancy Mental retardation Epilepsy (infantile spasms)	*Skin lesions:* Adenoma sebaceum (multiple tiny pink facial papules) Enlarge and coalesce Affect nose and cheek Onset ≈5 yrs age Irregular coarse (Shagreen) plaque Affects lumbosacral region Non-traumatic periungual fibroma ≥3 Hypopigmented oval (Ash) macules	

Moles

Diagnosis	Background	Key symptoms	Key signs	Additional information
Junctional naevus (Mole)	Immature melanocytes proliferate at dermo-epidermal junction Eventually migrate to dermis Commonly benign Typical onset in first 20 yrs Usually disappear with age Rarely become malignant	Acquired naevus Occurs anywhere on body No significant change in size No itching or bleeding	Single or multiple lesions Macular or slightly papular Round or oval Regular border Uniform pigmentation Light to dark brown colour Usually <7 mm diameter Gradually fades with time	A large number of melanocytic naevi and increased sun exposure increases risk of melanoma
Superficial capillary naevus (Stork mark)	Dilated capillaries of superficial dermis Commonly neonates Usually fades within 1 yr Neck lesions may persist	Occurs at birth Salmon-pink rash Affects: Glabellar, forehead, eyelids, nape Asymptomatic	Salmon-pink macular patch Usually fades	
Lentigo (pl. Lentigines)	Melanocyte proliferation and hyperpigmentation of epidermal basal layer			Some lentigines are associated with systemic syndromes
Common subtypes:				
Lentigo simplex	Commonest type Benign Congenital or acquired in childhood Not induced by sun exposure	Asymptomatic Occur anywhere on skin or mucous membranes Do not darken after sun exposure	Few in number Macular Round or oval Irregular or regular border Uniform pigmentation Brown to black colour Size 3–15 mm diameter Surrounded by normal skin	
Solar lentigo	Benign Sun-induced Commonly adults Affects fair skin types Usually reflects UV damage	Asymptomatic Affect sun-exposed areas: Shoulders, dorsum hands, face Slow increase in number and size Do not darken after sun exposure May darken with age	Multiple Macular or depressed Round or oval Uniform pigmentation Yellow–tan to black colour Initial size <5 mm diameter May coalesce to form a large patch Surrounded by normal skin	

Diagnosis	Background	Key symptoms	Key signs	Additional information
Infantile haemangioma ("Strawberry naevus")	Cavernous haemangioma Proliferative blood vessel tumour Benign Typical onset within first few days or first year of life Risk factors: Preterm and low birth weight infants Usually superficial Occasionally deep Most have resolved spontaneously by age 10 yrs	Common areas affected: Head and neck Usually asymptomatic Maximum growth within first 6 months Regression common after age >3 yrs	Usually solitary Dome-shaped nodule Dimpled surface Red–purple colour Easily bleeds on trauma	Earlier resoloution is associated with a better cosmetic result Subtle atrophy and telangiectasia may remain Refer complications: Airway/visual/auditory obstruction, haemorrhage, ulceration
Mongolian blue spot	Congenital Commonly Mongolian, South Asian and Afro-Carribeans Usually fades over the first year Occasionally persists	Blue–black patch Affects sacrum and buttocks Asymptomatic	Macular Diffuse Blue–black patch	
Deep capillary naevus (Port-wine stain)	Superficial capillary malformation Congenital Occasionally fades with time Most remain unchanged or deepen in colour	Deep pink or red patch Usually affects face or upper trunk Common in trigeminal area Gradually increases in size Often darkens with age	Usually unilateral Macular Irregular border Clearly circumscribed Deep pink, red or purple colour Variable size Normal overlying skin ± Surface papules (in adulthood)	An associated intracranial vascular malformation results in Sturg-Weber syndrome Congenital glaucoma can occur if ophthalmic division involved
Sutton's halo naevus	An immune response to a melanocytic naevus Benign Onset around puberty Usually resloves spontaneously over years	Asymptomatic brown naevus Commonly affects trunk No irritation, bleeding, ulceration	Single or multiple naevi Central uniformly pigmented naevus Round or oval in shape Followed by depigmentation of uniform width around the naevus ± Naevus involution ± Subsequent naevus repigmentation over years	
Common blue naevus	Deep dermal melanocytes Benign Typical onset in second decade Commonly Asians	Slate-grey or blue–black naevus Common areas: Scalp, neck, sacrum, dorsum hands/feet No change in size or shape	Solitary lesion Macular or papular Round shape Slate-grey or blue–black colour Size ≈2–7 mm diameter Smooth surface	Refer to exclude melanoma if increase in size or ulceration
Malignant melanoma	Risk factors: Chronic sun exposure, sunburn, sunbed use, multiple melanocytic naevi, Celtic skin, freckles, family history Age ≥15 yrs Spread via lymphatics and blood Metastasizes to lung, liver, brain Prognosis related to depth of tumour invasion		*Suspicious signs:* Rapid growth of a new mole in adults An old mole changing in shape and colour Irregular shape/border Uneven pigmentation (≥3 colours) New brown pigmented line of nail bed ± Bleeding ± Itching	Urgent dermatology referral
Subtypes:				
Superficial spreading melanoma 	Commonest melanoma Radial growth for months before vertical invasion	New or changing mole Common areas: Lower leg (women), back (men) or head/neck	Size ≥7 mm diameter Uneven pigmentation (brown, red, grey or black) Irregular shape/border	

Diagnosis	Background	Key symptoms	Key signs	Additional information
Nodular melanoma	Rapid growth Vertical invasion from the start Commonly older adults	Rapidly growing lump Commonly affects trunk	Initially flat pigmented lesion Irregular border Becomes nodular Bleeding or ulceration ± Warty surface	May also be non-pigmented (amelanotic)
Lentigo maligna melanoma	Develops from lentigo maligna (Hutchinson's freckle) Age >60 yrs Becomes invasive after many years Slow radial growth intially Followed by rapid vertical invasion	Increase in size of pre-existing lentigo maligna Commonly affects face	*Lentigo maligna:* Macular Irregular border Uneven brown pigmentation	Lentigo maligna is a patch of malignant melanocytes in sun-damaged skin. Usually proliferates radially for many years
Acral lentiginous melanoma	Not related to sun exposure Typical age 55–60 yrs Commonly Asian or Afro-Carribean	Affects: Soles, palms or subungual (thumb and big toenail)	Raised pigmented patch on soles/palms or New black–brown pigmented line of nail bed Extends to proximal and lateral nail fold ± Extension beyond nail	

Nail discolouration

Diagnosis	Background	Key symptoms	Key signs	Additional information
Nicotine staining	Chronic smoker	Gradual onset nail discolouration	Orange–brown nails Affects index and middle nail	
Tinea unguium **(Fungal nail infection)**	≈70% Trichophyton rubrum infection Initially infects epithelium nail bed Eventually spreads to nail plate Common in elderly >70 yrs age Risk factors: Immunosuppression, DM, humid climate, nail trauma, athletic/sporting activities, communal bathing, PVD	Affects finger and/or toe nail(s) ± Pain due to thickened nail	Creamy white or yellow nail Initially lateral nail bed affected Spreads proximally and/or across nail bed Thickened nail plate Subungual debris Onycholysis Distal nail friable on contact	Nail may not appear clear until months after treatment
Iron deficiency anaemia	Microcytic anaemia MCV <76 fl Causes: Chronic blood loss, poor diet, pregnancy, malabsorption	Breathless on exertion Fatigue Palpitations Chest pain	Pallor Koilonychia (spoon-shaped nails) Pale nails Glossitis Angular stomatitis	
Psoriasis (See Scales and Plaques)	Affects ≈50% of psoriatic patients Inflammation of proximal nail matrix Results in excess cells on nail surface As nail grows, cells are shed leaving pits and deformity	Nail deformity ± Cutaneous red plaque(s) with silvery scale	Creamy yellow nails Roughened appearance Surface pitting Brittle nails Subungual debris Onycholysis	Exclude fungal infection

Diagnosis	Background	Key symptoms	Key signs	Additional information
Chronic renal disease	Often end-stage renal failure patients on dialysis Independent of age	Nail discolouration	*Specific to ureamia:* Pink to brown discolouration of distal half of nail (Half-and-half) Affects single or multiple nails Fingers and/or toes ± Non-specific renal signs: Absent lunula Onycholysis Brittle nails Beau's lines on all nails (transverse nail grooves) Clubbing	
Leuconychia	Congenital or acquired Acquired causes: Fungal infection, cirrhosis, nephrotic syndrome, protein losing enteropathy, malnutrition, post-infection, lymphoma, minor nail trauma Associated with hypoalbuminaemia	Symptoms vary depending on underlying cause	White nails Either total, spots or striate form Often affects bilateral thumb and index nails ± Clubbing	
Splinter haemorrhages	Causes: Infective endocarditis, nail trauma, vasculitis (e.g. RA), haematological malignancy, severe anaemia	Symptoms vary depending on underlying cause	Red–purple linear streaks Parallel to long axis of nail Affects finger or toe nails	
Medication	Common drugs: Cytotoxic drugs, antimalarials, chlorpromazine, gold, tetracycline, minocycline	Onset after nail discolouration after taking medication Affects all nails	Nail discolouration varies depending on drug type	
Green nail syndrome	Pseudomonas infection Commonly found in soil, ground water, plants, animals Risk factors: Paronychia, frequent contact with water/detergents, nail/skin biting	Green–blue nail	Green–blue nail Fruity odour ± Paronchyia	
Yellow nail syndrome	Autosomal dominant No underlying nail infection Associated with bronchiectasis and lymphoedema	Slow nail growth	Blackish–yellow nails Thickened nail plate Increased curvature Onycholysis	
Acral lentiginous melanoma	Not related to sun exposure Typical age 55–60 yrs Commonly Asian or Afro-Carribean	Affects: Soles, palms, or subungual (thumb and big toenail)	New black–brown pigmented line of nail bed Extends to proximal and lateral nail fold ± Extension beyond nail	

Nodules*

Diagnosis	Background	Key symptoms	Key signs	Additional information
Boil (Furuncle)	Deep infection of a hair follicle Usually *Staphlococcus aureus* Common areas: Face, neck, armpits, buttocks, anogenital Usually self-limiting	Painful lump Gradually enlarges	Hard red epidermal nodule Surrounds hair follicle Tender on palpation Fluctuant Mobile ± Pus discharge from centre ± Inguinal LN	Infection of adjacent hair follicles (carbuncle), fever or cellulitis warrants antibiotics

*Nodule: a circumscribed visible or palpable lump >0.5 cm

Diagnosis	Background	Key symptoms	Key signs	Additional information
Sebaceous cyst (Epidermoid cyst)	Proliferation of epidermal cells in the dermis Benign Slow growth Commonly young adults M>F Common sites: Face, trunk, neck, extremities, scalp Often resolves spontaneously Usually recurs if not excised	Painless lump(s)	Single or multiple Skin coloured Often round or oval Variable in size Firm subcutaneous nodule Central punctum Fixed to skin Not reducible Not pulsatile ± Uninfected foul cheese-like discharge	A tender and erythematous cyst suggests infection
Lipoma	Adipose tumour Usually benign Slow growth Commonly adults Often multiple (lipomatosis) Common sites: Neck, trunk, upper arms, shoulders Does not occur on palms or soles Can occur in deeeper tissues	Painless lump(s)	Single or multiple Skin coloured Often irregular in shape Usually <5 cm diameter Soft subcutaneous nodule Smooth normal skin surface Mobile Not reducible Not pulsatile	If >5 cm and rapid growth, refer to exclude liposarcoma
Warts	Benign epidermal neoplasm Caused by HPV Spread by direct or indirect contact Risk factors: Skin abrasion, frequent wet work with hands, hyperhidrosis of feet, swimming pools, nail biting ≈65% spontaneously disappear within 2 yrs No associated scarring			Warts often persist and recur if immunocompromised
Subtypes:				
Common warts	Commonly school-aged children and young adults	Usually affect hands and knees ± Painful	Single or grouped Raised cauliflower-like nodules Irregular papillomatous surface Firm Variable size Scatter, cluster or periungual distribution	
Plane warts		Usually affects face and dorsum of hands	Single or grouped May coalesce Slightly raised papules Size 0.2–0.4 cm diameter Flat-topped smooth surface Skin coloured ± Linear distribution along scratches/abrasions	
Plantar warts		Usually affects soles of feet Painful	Small area of thickened skin Keratinised surface Underlying black dots (thrombosed capillaries) Solitary, scatter or grouped (mosaic) distribution	

Diagnosis	Background	Key symptoms	Key signs	Additional information
Basal cell carcinoma	Insidious growth Locally destructive Commonly age >30 yrs Risk factors: Celtic/fair skin, sun exposure Rarely metastatic			All types may be unevenly pigmented
Common subtypes:				
Nodular-ulcerative BCC (Rodent ulcer) 	Commonly affects head and neck	New onset papule becomes nodular Slow growth over months/years Often painless Bleeding on contact Fails to heal	Nodular lesion Pearlescent pink colour Telangiectatic surface ± Depressed ulcerating centre ± "Pearly" rolled edge	
Superficial BCC 	Affects head, neck, trunk, limbs	New onset plaque Slow growth over years ± Bleeding or weeping	Typically solitary Scaly erythematous plaque Raised "worm-like" edge Well demarcated	
Morphoeic BCC	Aggressive BCC	"Scar-like" lesion	Grey or yellow plaque Poorly defined border Variable size	
Eruptive xanthomas	Cutaneous lipd-laden histiocytes Indicates hypertriglyceridaemia Risk factors: Familial hyperlipidaemia, IHD, DM, alcohol abuse, chronic renal disease, hypothyroidism, PBC, monoclonal gammopathies, drugs (e.g. beta-blockers, diuretics)	Acute onset skin papules or nodules Common sites: Eyelids (Xanthelasma), extensor surfaces of limbs, tendons, palmar creases ± Mildly tender and/or itchy	Crops of yellow papules or nodules Erythematous base	Resolution with treatment of underlying cause
Dermatofibroma	Benign skin tumour Commonly young adults M:F ratio: ≈1:4 Usually persists indefinitely	Commonly affects lower legs Typically asymptomatic No change in size	Single or multiple Skin-coloured or pink/red or creamy/brown nodule Round Size 0.5–1.0 cm diameter Firm to hard texture Feels "like a lentil" Mobile Smooth surface Squeezing sides causes surface dimpling	

Diagnosis	Background	Key symptoms	Key signs	Additional information
Squamous cell carcinoma	Malignant More common in Caucasions Incidence increases with age Risk factors: Chronic UV exposure, genital HPV infection, immunosupression, chemical or radiation exposure, pre-cancerous lesions (e.g. actinic keratoses)	Typically affects sun-exposed areas: Scalp, face, pinna, lower lip, back, chest, lower legs Non-healing ulcer or rapidly growing polypoid mass	Shallow ulcer Rolled edges Overlying plaque Or polypoid mass ± Localised LN *High-risk signs:* Periauricular or lip lesions Size >2 cm diameter Depth >0.4 cm	Exclude cranial nerve involvment in facial lesions Urgent skin biopsy
Rheumatoid nodules	Commonest exra-articular manifestation of RA May affect internal organs (e.g. lungs, heart) Suggests sero-positive RA and severe disease Also associated with non-rheumatoid conditions (e.g. SLE) May grow or regress with time High recurrence rate	Affect pressure points: Forearms, elbows, dorsum hands, feet Non-tender nodules	Skin-coloured nodules Subcutaneous Size 0.2 cm to >5 cm Firm on palpation Mobile or fixed to underlying tissue	Complications: Pain, joint immobility, deformity, erosion, infection
Heberden's nodes	Calcific spurs of articular cartilage Indicate nodular osteoarthritis Age >50 yrs M:F ratio: ≈1:10 Predominantly Caucasion	History of acute or chronic joint sweling Followed by: Painful swelling of DIP joints Joint morning stiffness ≤30 mins Also worse after activity ± PIP joint involvement ± Carpometacarpal thumb joint involvement	*Nodular joint formation:* Asymmetrical node formation Affects DIP joints Firm or bony nodules Joint tenderness and swelling Warmth Limited joint movement ± Bouchard nodes over PIP joints	
Keratoacanthoma	Low-grade malignant nodule Originates in pilosebaceous glands Commonly elderly age >60 yrs M:F ratio: ≈2:1 Risk factors include: UV exposure, chemical carcinogens Rarely invasive or metastatic Slow spontaneous resolution within 4–12 months with scarring	Acute onset nodule Affects sun-exposed areas Rapid growth over weeks	Usually solitary Skin coloured or reddish Round dome-shaped nodule Well circumscribed Rolled edges Central crater of keratin or ulceration Smooth shiny surface Erythematous and inflamed base	Exclude squamous cell carcinoma
Gouty tophi	Chronic gout and hyperuricaemia Crystal (tophaceous) deposits of sodium urate Affects: Soft tissue, bone, tendons Causes joint damage and deformity	Often history of gout >10 yrs Painless nodule(s) Typically affects: Extensor surfaces of hand, forearm, elbow, Achilles tendon, pinna	Asymmetrical large nodules Non-tender Irregular and firm texture Chalky appearance beneath skin Limited joint movement ± Ulceration and discharge	
Chondrodermatitis nodularis helicis	Inflammatory nodule Benign M>F Commonly affects right > left ear Likely risk factors: Skin trauma, inflammation, sun/cold damage	Acute onset symptoms Painful nodule on external ear Worse with pressure (e.g. sleep) Nodule grows for a few months Followed by static growth	Usually solitary Skin-coloured nodule on helix Round or oval Well circumscribed Size 0.5–2 cm diameter Firm texture Raised rolled edge Erythematous edge ± Central necrosis or collagen	
Keloid scar	Overgrowth of dense fibrous tissue Extends beyond borders of original wound Can occur spontaneously Highest incidence in Sub-Saharan Africans Risk factors: Skin cuts, ear-piercings, burns, acne, BCG innoculations	Often history of skin trauma Initially raised red lesion Itchy Usually grows slowly over months to years ± Painful	Raised nodular lesion Extends beyond boundaries of original wound Brown or pale colour with age Round, oval or oblong Regular or irregular border Flat or pedunculated surface Soft or rubbery texture No hair follicles	Keloids over a joint can contract and thus restrict movement

Diagnosis	Background	Key symptoms	Key signs	Additional information
Pyogenic granuloma	Reactive inflammatory mass of capillaries and fibroblasts Benign Commonly children age 6–7 yrs and pregnancy Common risk factors: Skin trauma or infection Lesions in pregnancy often regress spontaneously after childbirth	Acute onset new nodule Commonly affects digits and gums Rapid growth over weeks Easily bleeds on contact ± History of skin trauma/infection	Solitary nodule Red, purple or yellow colour Arises from normal skin Polypoid Variable size Friable: Bleeding, ulcerated or crusted	
Nodular melanoma (See Moles)				
Neurofibromatosis Type 1 (See Hyperpigmentation)				

Papules

Diagnosis	Background	Key symptoms	Key signs	Additional information
Acne vulgaris (See Facial erythema)				
Skin tag **(Acrochordon)**	Benign Commonly affects elderly Risk factors: Advancing age and obesity	Often catch on clothing Commonly affects: Skin folds (e.g. neck, axillae, eyelids)	Single or multiple Skin-coloured or brown papules Pedunculated lesions Size 0.2–0.5 cm	
Molluscum contagiosum 	Caused by Poxvirus Commonly children with atopic eczema Spread by direct contact Typically spontaneous resolution occurs in 6–9 months	Non-itchy papules Common areas: Head, neck, trunk	Grouped papules Pearly white colour Shiny surface Central umbilication Size 0.5–1.0 cm diameter ± Crusting and suppuration on healing ± Surrounding patchy eczema	
Urticaria **(Wheals)**	Dermal oedema and vasodilatation Causes: Idiopathic, IgE, mast cell activation, autoimmune, drugs No scarring			Airway compromise warrants adrenaline and emergency admission Individual wheals lasting >24 h may reflect an underlying sytemic disease
Subtypes:				
Acute urticaria	Attacks lasts <6 wks duration Triggers: Plants, food (e.g. nuts, shellfish), drugs (e.g. aspirin) Each wheal lasts for <24 h Associated with atopy	Acute onset wheals Initially white papules then pink with white rim Generalised distribution Intense pruritis Burning	Multiple papules Blanching pink colour Variable size and shape ± Angioedema	
Chronic idiopathic urticaria	Attacks last >6 wks Multiple triggers (e.g. chronic ingestion of food colourings Each wheal lasts for <24 h	Gradual onset wheals As above	As above	
Physical urticaria	Triggered by physical insults Common triggers: Scratching (dermatographism), pressure, sweat, cold, water, UV exposure, heat	Acute or gradual onset wheals As above	As above	

Diagnosis	Background	Key symptoms	Key signs	Additional information
Campbell de Morgan spot	Angiomas Develop during adult life Benign Commonly middle-age or older Increase in frequency and size with age Does not affect mucous membranes	Asymptomatic papules Commonly affect trunk and extremities Papules may grow with time	Multiple small papules Cherry red or violaceous colour Size ≈0.1–0.3 cm Non-blanching	
Miliaria ("Prickly heat")	Due to sweat obstruction Commonly neonates	Tiny red papules Affect: Face, trunk, napkin area Pruritis Worse with hot weather Relieved with skin cooling	Crops of red papules	
Scabies	Female scabies mite infestation Obligate human parasite Forms epidermal burrows and lays eggs Life span 4–6 wks Risk factors: Overcrowding, social deprivation Spread via prolonged physical contact Pruritis can persist for 3 wks post successful treatment	Onset symptoms >4 wks post-infection Intense pruritis Worse at night	*Burrows:* Tortuous lines 0.2–1.5 cm long Silvery-grey colour Vesicle at closed end of burrow Excoriation marks Common areas: Hand/feet webspaces, flexures, male genitals Or face and neck in children ± Vesicles or crusts *Allergic rash:* Symmetrical Erythematous papules Commonly affects: Peri-umbilicus, axillae, buttocks ± Secondary infection	Close contacts should be simultaneously treated Occasionally hyper-infestation (Crusted "Norwegian" scabies) occurs in those who are immunosuppressed and/or unable to scratch
Milia	Keratin-filled cysts Common in all ages including newborns Can be familial	Spontaneous onset or History of skin trauma or blistering Common on cheeks or around eyes ± Palate (Epstein pearls) Asymptomatic	Multiple tiny papules Superficial Pearly white to yellowish colour Size 0.1–0.2 cm diameter Uniform dome-shaped	
Keratosis pilaris	Hair follicles become blocked with horny plugs of keratin Commonly adolescents M<F ≈50% are familial Often resolves spontaneously over years	Commonly affects: Cheeks, upper outer arm, anterior thighs, buttocks Affected skin feels rough ± Pruritis	Multiple red papular projections Around hair follicles ± Erythematous base Size 0.1–0.2 cm diameter Roughened skin appearance	
Localised granuloma annulare	Benign inflammatory condition Age <30 yrs M:F ratio: ≈1:2 Usually resolve spontaneously within 2 yrs Can recur	Commonly affects: Dorsum hands/feet, elbows, ankles ± Pain on trivial injury	Well-defined annular plaques Surrounded by skin-coloured papules Size 0.1–0.2 cm diameter Firm texture ± Hyperpigmented sunken centre	

Diagnosis	Background	Key symptoms	Key signs	Additional information
Guttate psoriasis 	Common presentation of psoriasis in young adults Associated with: Streptococcal throat infection, stress, skin trauma, drugs (e.g. antimalarials, NSAID) Usually self-limiting within a few weeks Can progress to stable plaques	History of recent throat infection Acute eruption of papules Affects: Trunk and proximal extremities Mildy pruritis	Multiple drop-like papules Salmon-pink colour Size ≈1cm diameter Fine scaly surface ± Nail pitting	
Lichen planus 	Immune-mediated Associated with PBC Spontaneous resolution of cutaneous lesions usually within 2 yrs Oral lesions are often persistent Small risk of malignant change	Acute onset symptoms Intensely itchy papules Affects: Wrists, ankles, dorsum hands, buccal mucosa, genitals, scars (Koebner phenomenon)	Multiple papules Violaceous colour Size 0.2–0.5 cm diameter Round Flat-topped White surface lines (Wickham's striae) ± Nail changes *Oral lichen planus:* Slightly raised mucosal streaks Lacy appearance ± Pain	
Orf	Caused by a parapox virus Endemic in sheep and goats Spread via direct animal–human contact Incubation 5–6 days Spontaneous resolution within 3–6 wks Lifelong immunity	Asymptomatic lesion Commonly affects fingers and forearms	Often a solitary lesion Initially a papule Rapidly becomes a granulomatous nodule Variable size ± Ulceration	Complications: Erythema multiforme and lymphadenitis
Lyme disease	Tick-borne illness Caused by *Borellia burgdorferi* Transmitted by Ixodid tick vectors Peaks in spring and summer Ticks common in deers Bites enlarge to form erythema chronica migrans Symptoms usually settle within 4 wks Skin rash may persist	*Initial stage:* Red skin bites Affects: Groin, thigh, axilla *Early stage: days to weeks later* Fatigue Headache Stiff neck Arthralgia Myalgia	*Initial stage:* Red macule/papule (tick bites) *Early stage: days to weeks later* Erythema chronicum migrans (hot painless annular lesion) Fever Lymphadenopathy Hepatomegaly ± Secondary skin lesions (e.g. malar rash)	Failure to treat early stage leads to multi-system involvement months later (e.g. pericarditis, arthritis, meningitis)
Tuberous sclerosis (See Hypopigmentation)				
Secondary syphilis (See Vulval lump or ulcer)				

Petechiae and ecchymoses*

Diagnosis	Background	Key symptoms	Key signs	Additional information
Trauma	History of minor or major physical trauma	Tender bruises Not recurrent	Localised bruises	Children can develop petechiae around eyes following vigorous coughing or vomiting Consider NAI if multiple bruises of varying age in a person who is otherwise well

Purpura: Red/purplish bleeding beneath skin
Petechiae: Purpura <1 cm diameter
*Ecchymoses: Purpura >1 cm diameter

Diagnosis	Background	Key symptoms	Key signs	Additional information
Senile purpura	Elderly Normal clotting	Recurrent bruising Due to minor trauma Common areas: Dorsum of hands and limbs No malaise	Systemically well Widespread bruises Dark purple colour Non-tender No petechiae	
Medication	Common drugs: Heparin, warfarin, chronic steroid use Adverse drug reactions may cause blood dyscrasias	Onset of bruising after taking medication	Widespread bruising Non-tender No petechiae	
Cirrhosis (See Jaundice)				
Allergic vasculitis **(Leukocystoclastic vasculitis)**	Acute or chronic Small-vessel vasculitis Can be cutaneous only or Extracutaneous (e.g. kidneys, GIT) and joints Possible triggers: Drugs (e.g. amoxicillin), bacterial/viral infections, hepatitis C, IBD, collagen diseases	Purpuric rash Typically on lower legs ± Pruritis, burning sensation or pain ± Systemic symptoms vary depending on organs involved: Arthralgia Myalgia Abdominal pain Haematuria	Multiple palpable purpura Size 1–3 mm diameter May coalesce to form plaques or Become haemorrhagic vesicles or bullae	
Henoch-Schönlein purpura	Commonest allergic vasculitis IgA-mediated Small-vessel vasculitis Affects: Kidneys, abdomen, skin Commonly 3–10 yrs age M:F ratio: ≈2:1 Often follows recent URTI Usually self-limiting within several weeks	Skin rash Lower-limb arthralgia Colicky abdominal pain Vomiting Diarrhoea (can be bloody) Haematuria	Mild fever Symmetrical purpuric rash ± Slightly raised Non-itchy Affects buttocks and back of legs Swollen tender lower-limb joints *Abnormal urinalysis:* Haematuria Proteinuria	Renal complications are more frequent and severe in older children
Leukaemia	Causes thrombocytopenic purpura			
Subtypes:				
Acute myeloid leukaemia	Myeloid stem cells arrest in early development Abnormal proliferation of cells Infiltration of bone marrow, blood, organs Class of AML dependent on cell type Commonly affects adults Incidence increases up to age 50 yrs Risk factors: Aplastic anaemia, myelofibrosis, polycythaemia rubra vera, CLL, previous cytotoxic chemotherapy	Acute or chronic symptoms Spontaneous bruising Bleeding gums Fatigue Shortness of breath Bony pain	Fever Anaemia Petechiae Gingivitis Hepatosplenomegaly ± Bruises ± Pneumonia	
Acute lymphoblastic leukaemia	Malignant lymphoid precursors Usually B-cells Infiltration of bone marrow and blood Peak in children age 2–4 yrs and adults >50 yrs Risk factors: Genetic, radiation exposure	History of recurrent infections Spontaneous bruising Epistaxis Fatigue Shortness of breath Severe bony pain including joints	Tachycardia Anaemia Petechiae Gingivitis Local or generalised LN Abdominal distension Hepatosplenomegaly Testicular enlargement ± Bruises	Children generally have a better prognosis
Chronic lymphocytic leukaemia	Malignancy of B-lymphocytes Commonly age >55 yrs Possible genetic predisposition High WCC can cause hyperviscosity syndrome	Insidious onset symptoms Spontaneous bruising Fatigue Recurrent infection (e.g. pneumonia, herpes simplex)	Anaemia Petechiae Local or generalised LN Hepatosplenomegaly ± Bruises	A major cause of death is secondary malignancy

Diagnosis	Background	Key symptoms	Key signs	Additional information
Chronic myeloid leukaemia	Abnormal proliferation of haemopoietic stem cell line(s) Commonly age >60 yrs Associated with Philadelphia chromosome Quiescent for years before rapid onset of myeloproliferation	Insidious onset symptoms Spontaneous bruising Fatigue Weight loss Night sweats Abdominal fullness LUQ pain (splenic infarction)	Fever Anaemia Petechiae Local or generalised LN Abdominal distension Hepatosplenomegaly Gout (rapid cell turnover) Hyperviscosity syndrome (e.g. CVA) ± Bruises	
Thrombocytopenia				
Common subtypes:				
Idiopathic	IgG antibodies destroy platelets In children M = F Often self-limiting in children following viral infection Can be chronic in young adults M:F ratio: ≈1:3	Often acute onset symptoms Prolonged, excessive or recurrent nosebleeds Bleeding gums Spontaneous bruising ± Haemoptysis ± Haematemesis ± Blood in stool	Generalised petechiae Bruises	Splenomegaly or lymphadenopathy suggest a more sinister cause (e.g. marrow failure)
Alloimmune	History of blood transfusion Occurs 10 days to several months post-transfusion	As above	As above	
Drug induced	Drugs include: Warfarin, ibuprofen, carbamezapine, amiodarone, cimetidine, ranitidine, phenytoin, heparin, alcohol	As above	As above	
Meningitis (See Headache)				
Disseminated intravascular coagulation	Rapid consumption of clotting factors results in haemorrhage Thrombocytopenia and low fibrinogen levels Triggered by underlying pathology (e.g. septicaemia, leukaemia) Subacute or chronic DIC are asssociated with venous thrombosis	Symptoms vary depending on underlying pathology	Fever Confusion Spontaneous bleeding (e.g. i.v. sites) Generalised petechiae Generalised bruising ± Thrombosis	

Pustules

Diagnosis	Background	Key symptoms	Key signs	Additional information
Non-bullous impetigo	Superficial skin infection Group A Streptococci and/or *Staphylococcus aureus* infection Commonly school-aged children More prevalent in summer Highly contagious via skin contact Rapid spread Risk factors: Eczema, allergic dermatitis, grazed skin Scarring is uncommon	Painless itchy pustules Affects any part of the body Commonly affects face	Tiny superficial pustules or vesicles Surrounding skin is erythematous Lesions rupture easily Scab over with golden crust Moist and erythematous skin Regional LN	School exclusion until lesions have crusted and healed In severe and recurrent staphylococcal infection consider DM

Diagnosis	Background	Key symptoms	Key signs	Additional information
Folliculitis	Infection of superficial hair follicle Commonly *Staphylococcus aureus* Pseudomonas infection associated with hot tubs and pools Risk factors: Thick hair, shaving "against grain" skin friction, hyperhydrosis, atopic eczema, immunocompromise, chronic topical steroids, skin abrasion, nasal carriage of S. Aureus	Gradual onset red skin lumps Affects hair-borne areas Pruritis	Small discrete pustules Centred on hair follicle Erythematous base	In severe and recurrent staphylococcal infection consider DM
Acne vulgaris (See Facial erythema)				
Acne rosacea (See Facial erythema)				
Perioral dermatitis	Chronic facial dermatitis Commonly women aged 20–45 yrs Associated with use of topical steroids	Episodes of circumoral erythema Worse after stopping steroids or exposure to UV light, wind, heat Burning sensation Rarely itchy Common areas: Circumoral, nasolabial folds, lateral portion of lower lids	Groups of small papules, vesicles and pustules On an erythematous base Circumoral pallor	Withdrawal of topical steroids often causes an intial worsening of symptoms
Cutaneous Candidiasis	Commonly *Candida albicans* Yeast infection Normal commensal of the gut Affects: Mucous membranes, nails, genitals and skin			
Common subtypes:				
Angular cheilitis (Angular stomatitis)	Infection of deep skin creases of the mouth corners due to constant moist skin Infective causes: Candida or staphylococci Risk factors: Sagging facial muscles, ill-fitting dentures	Sore corners of the mouth Burning sensation	Erythema at the mouth corners Maceration ± Pustules and crusting (if secondary bacterial infection)	Consider iron and/or vitamin B deficiency
Intertrigo	Risk factors: Obesity, poor hygiene, humidity, DM, previous seborrhoeic dermatitis	Burning sensation Pruritis Affects skin apposition surfaces: Submammary, axillae, groin	Maceration and weeping skin Patchy erythema Creamy satellite pustules at the margin Easily rupture leaving a collarette of scale	
Hidradenitis suppurativa	Chronic relapsing suppurative disease Affects apocrine glands Commonly age 20–30 yrs M<F Associated with severe acne	Skin nodule Pruritis Painful Persists for weeks/months Nodule develops into a pustule Ruptures with purulent pus Areas affected: Axillae, groin, submammary, perineum	Solitary or multiple nodule(s) Localised or scattered Superficial or subcutaneous Recurrent pustular formation Chronic discharge (purulent/bloody)	Complications include internal fistula formation
Pyoderma gangrenosum	Ulcerating skin condition Skin trauma may induce new lesions (Pathergy) No underlying infection Typically 30–40 yrs age Associated with: IBD, arthritis, myeloma Residual scarring	Initially lesion is a papule or pustule with surrounding erythema Pustule grows in size Gradually becomes necrotic Painful Classically affects legs ± Malaise ± Arthralgia	Solitary or multiple lesions Deep ulcer Violaceous border Well demarcated ± Fever	Complications include secondary infection

Diagnosis	Background	Key symptoms	Key signs	Additional information
Palmoplantar pustulosis	Acute or chronic condition Plaque psoriasis often co-exists Commonly age 20–60 yrs M<F Risk factors: Smoking and family history	Red palms and/or soles Superficial pustules Uncomfortable or painful No pruritis	Systemically well Unilateral or bilateral Erythematous palms and/or soles Thickened fissured skin Scaly appearance Crops of superficial sterile pustules Gradually become brown and scaly Eventually peel off	
Pustular psoriasis	Possible history of psoriasis	Acute onset widespread erythema Tender skin Eruption of clusters and papules Pustules coalesce and dry out New pustules occur for days/weeks Chills Malaise Nausea Arthralgia	High-grade swinging fever >39°C Tachypnoea Tachycardia Generalised sterile pustules Size 1–3 mm in diameter Erythematous skin	

Scales and plaques

Diagnosis	Background	Key symptoms	Key signs	Additional information
Psoriasis	Chronic relapsing condition Epidermal hyperproliferation and accumulation of inflammatory cells Commonly Caucasians Risk factors: Genetic, infection, skin trauma, drugs (e.g. beta-blockers), alcohol abuse, emotional stress, smoking	Worse in winter Improves in summer		Different subtypes may co-exist
Common subtypes:				
Classical plaque psoriasis	Commonest subtype Chronic stable plaques Can occur at the site of scars/trauma (Köebner phenomenon) Can resolve spontaneously	Scaly plaque(s) Pruritis Common on extensor surfaces: Knees, elbows, sacrum Flexures and face in children ± Plaques enlarge slowly ± Coalesce with other plaques	Solitary or mulitple plaques Red colour Symmetrical distribution Irregular or oval shape Variable size Thin silvery-white scaly surface Erythematous friable base ± Nail pitting (See Nail discoloration) ± Arthropathy in up to 20%	
Scalp psoriasis		Thick scaly scalp	Solitary or multiple plaques Palpable thick silvery-white scale Erythematous friable base ± Thick clumps of scale on hair ± Temporary hair loss	

Diagnosis	Background	Key symptoms	Key signs	Additional information
Guttate psoriasis	Common presentation of psoriasis in young adults Associated with: Streptococcal throat infection, stress, skin trauma, drugs (e.g. antimalarials, NSAID) Usually self-limiting within a few weeks Can progress to stable plaques	History of recent throat infection Acute eruption of papules Affects trunk and proximal extremities Mild pruritis	Multiple drop-like papules Salmon-pink colour Size ≈1 cm diameter Fine scaly surface ± Nail pitting	
Flexural psoriasis		Red rash Pruritis Common areas: Natal cleft, groin, axillae, umbilicus, submammary folds	Beefy erthematous patches Maceration No scaly plaques	
Brittle psoriasis	May occur de novo or may develop from stable plaque psoriasis Risk factors: Systemic or topical steroid use	Red inflamed skin	Erythematous areas Scaly surface No plaques	May rapidly generalise to form erythroderma or acute pustular psoriasis
Erythroderma (Exfoliative dermatitis)	Loss of thermoregulation Water and protein loss from skin	Acute onset symptoms Widespread red inflamed skin Shivering	Generalised erythema Scaly surface Hot skin on palpation Generalised LN	Admit immediately Risk of cardiac failure, renal failure, hypothermia
Infant seborrhoeic dermatitis (Cradle cap)	Affects sebum-rich areas Associated with Malassezia furfur Small risk of adult seborrhoeic dermatitis <10% Often resolves spontaneously in 12–24 months	Onset a few weeks post-partum Flaky patches of skin or plaque Affects scalp Scalp not itchy ± Itchy erythema in the nappy area	Well child Yellow scaling patches on scalp Greasy appearance Surrounding erythema ± Partial loss of hair ± Flexural erythema in nappy area ± Plaques around eyebrows, ears, nose	Beware secondary infection in excoriated lesions
Seborrhoeic dermatitis (See Facial erythema)				
Atopic eczema (Atopic dermatitis)	Chronic relapsing condition Typical onset <2 yrs age Causes: Genetic (FH atopy), allergic component (e.g. IgE), environmental allergens (e.g. animal dander) Associated with allergic rhinitis and asthma Childhood eczema often resolves by early teens	Intensely itchy dry skin Generalised in early stages Localises to flexures later Common areas: Neck, wrists, antecubital and popliteal fossae	Patches of diffuse erythema Local skin oedema Prominent skin creases Dry scaling surface Thickened skin (lichenification) Fissures Vesicles	Common complications: Folliculitis, impetigo, warts, Molluscum contagiosum
Seborrhoeic wart (Seborrhoeic keratosis)	Benign hyperkeratotic lesions Commonly age >50 yrs Risk factors: Familial and UV exposure	Typically asymptomatic Initially a hyperpigmented macule Gradually becomes a plaque Grows and becomes thicker with time Affects: Head, neck, trunk, dorsum of hands, forearms ± Can become inflamed or itchy after minor trauma	Single or multiple Deeply pigmented brown–black Well circumscribed Up to 3 cm in diameter Flat-topped plaques "Stuck on" warty appearance Irregular pitted greasy surface	

Diagnosis	Background	Key symptoms	Key signs	Additional information
Actinic keratoses (Solar keratoses) 	Dysplastic squamous epithelium Not invasive Pre-malignant Many clinical variants Incidence increases with age Risk factors: Fair skinned, excess UV exposure	Red scaly patches Wax and wane with time Bleed easily with minor trauma Affects sun-exposed areas: Face, bald scalp, forearms, dorsum hands, helical rims	Multiple discrete lesions Variable size Erythematous base Scaly surface (hyperkeratosis) Some become thicker than others Feels rough	Larger (>10 mm) multiple lesions have a higher risk of developing SCC
Tinea infection	Common fungi: Trichophytons, Microsporum, Epidermophyton Invades and grows in dead keratin Encouraged by warmth and moisture Spread from humans or animals			
Common subtypes:				
Tinea unguium (See Nail discolouration)				
Tinea pedis (Athlete's foot)	Dermatophyte infection of the feet Risk factors: Communal swimming pools, showers	Itchy toe-webs and/or soles Rash spreads across the foot	Asymmetrical Scaling surface ± Erythema ± Vesicles and pustules	
Tinea cruris	Commonly men Feet are typically infected also	Ring-like rash Pruritis Affects groin ± Perineum and buttocks	Annular erythematous patches Raised erythematous margin Scaly surface Central clearing Gradually enlarges	
Tinea capitis (See Hair loss)				
Tinea corporis 	Common source of infection: Feet in adults and scalp in children	Ring-like rash Pruritis Affects trunk and limbs	Annular erythematous patches Raised erythematous margin Scaly surface Central clearing Gradually becomes confluent	
Pityriasis versicolor (See Hypopigmentation)				
Pityriasis rosea	Typically children and young adults Common in spring and autumn Self-limiting within 6–8 wks ± Hypo/hyperpigmentation post-rash	Mild prodomal symptoms may present first Followed by ≥1 "herald" patches Intense pruritis Affects: Neck, trunk or proximal limbs Rash becomes generalised days later	"Herald patch": Large round or oval plaque(s) Central wrinkled salmon colour Dark-red margin Fine scaly margin (peripheral collarette) Size 1–2 cm diameter Followed by secondary rash separate from original herald patch: Symmetrical Multiple small herald patches Truncal Christmas tree distribution Oral lesions are rare	Atypical variant includes a peripheral rash, facial rash in children and blisters

Diagnosis	Background	Key symptoms	Key signs	Additional information
Discoid lupus erythematosus	Usually no systemic involvement Commonly age 20–40 yrs M:F ratio: ≈1:2 Lesions heal with scarring Malignant change is rare SLE more likely to develop in generalised lesions	Usually asymptomatic or Erythematous plaques Gradually enlarge Affects: Scalp, face, neck, dorsum hands, arms ± Buccal and/or nasal mucosa involvement worse after sun exposure	Multiple active plaques May coalesce Erythematous Irregular hyperpigmented margin Shiny hypopigmented atrophic centre Scaly surface Follicular plugging	Scalp lesions may be associated with permanent alopecia
Bowen's disease 	Squamous cell carcinoma in situ Commonly age 60–70 yrs Risk factors: Fair skin, chronic UV exposure, immunocompromise	Asymptomatic or Red or pink patch of skin Slow growing Typically affects sun-exposed areas	Usually solitary plaque Red or pink colour Well demarcated Variable size Scaly adherent surface Non-friable base	Can affect the glans penis (Erythroplasia of Queyrat)
Lichen simplex chronicus	Localised form of atopic eczema Typical age 30–50 yrs Causes: Eczema, scars, insect bites, venous insufficiency	History of focal scratching/rubbing Localised plaque Intense pruritus Common areas: Shins, forearms, nape, genitalia	Solitary plaque Reddish purple colour Well demarcated Size >5 cm diameter Thickened skin (lichenification) Excoriation marks Scaly surface	
Juvenile plantar dermatosis	Due to synthetic socks and shoes Exacerbated by sweating and friction Commonly children age 4–8 yrs M>F More prevalent in summer	Painful soles of feet	Dry scaly and peeling skin Shiny red surface Painful fissures Affects weight-bearing areas Normal skin in toe-webs	
Ichthyosis vulgaris	Hyperkeratosis of horny skin layer Due to excess keratin Typical age >1 yr Autosomal dominant Normally improves with age Associated with atopy	Extremely dry and flaky skin Affects: Face, trunk, extensor surfaces of limbs Worse in cold weather Relieved in warm weather	Dry and scaly skin Fine white surface "cracks" Hyperkeratosis of palms and soles Keratosis pilaris (See Papules) Limb flexures usually not affected	
Morphoea	Sclerosis (thickening) of the skin No systemic involvement Commonly young adults M<F Gradual spontaneous resolution Residual hyperpigmentation	Initially mauve plaques Gradually become ivory colour after months Plaques do not sweat	Solitary or multiple plaques Ivory colour Iliac margin Size 1 to ≥20 cm diameter Indurated Shiny smooth surface Hairless	
Subtypes:				
Circumscribed	Commonest subtype	Common on trunk	As above	
Linear	Can impair limb growth in childhood	Usually affects one entire limb	Linear narrow plaque ± Flexion contracture	
Frontoparietal (En coupe de sabre)	A significant cosmetic problem May cause skull bone shrinkage	Affects face and scalp	Linear narrow plaque Indurated and depressed Extends from face to scalp Permanent hair loss along the plaque	

Diagnosis	Background	Key symptoms	Key signs	Additional information
Generalised		Affects trunk and limbs	Generalised sclerosis ± Flexion contractures ± Limited limb movement	
Cutaneous T-cell lymphoma (Mycosis fungoides)	Primary cutaneous lymphoma ≈65% are T-cell type Commonest type: Mycosis fungoides Typical age 40–60 yrs Low grade/slow growing Remains localised to skin for years	Affects any part of body *Patch stage:* Lasts for years Red skin patches May disappear spontaneously, remain unchanged or grow slowly ± Pruritis *Plaque stage:* Patches gradually become thicker Pruritis *Tumour stage:* Plaques become lumpy	*Patch stage:* Lasts for years Multiple flat patches Red colour Oval or annular shape Well circumscribed Scaly surface *Plaque stage:* Thick scaly plaques Well circumscribed *Tumour stage:* Large irregular nodules ± Ulceration ± Metastasis	Refer for skin biospy Early patches may mimic eczema or psoriasis
Kaposi's sarcoma	Malignant vascular tumour Caused by Herpes virus Type 8 Many types of KS Classical (indolent) KS common in the immunocompetent Aggressive KS more common in immunodeficient M>F *Risk factors:* Male gender, Ashkenazi Jews, Mediterraneans, Africans, immunodeficiency (e.g. AIDS)	*Classical KS:* Commonly affects legs Slow progression over years Usually no pruritis Usually painless *Transplant/aquired KS:* Commonly affects: Mouth, nose, throat Rapid dissemination Usually no pruritis Usually painless	Solitary or multiple lesions Plaques and/or nodular lesions Red–purplish or black colour ± Metastasis	Urgent referral

Chapter 11
Mental Health

Abnormal behaviour

Diagnosis	Background	Key symptoms	Key signs	Additional information
Alcohol intoxication	Commonly teenagers and young adults	History of alcohol abuse	Smell of alcohol Slurred speech Facial flushing Unsteady gait Nystagmus Limb incoordination Aggressive or disinhibited behaviour	Beware of coexisting head injury or hypoglycaemia as a true cause of confusion
Acute confusional state (Delirium) (See Acute confusion)	Common in hospitalised patients Typically elderly Causes: Infection, MI, hypoxia, hypoglycaemia, electrolyte abnormality, DKA, CVA, medication overdose, head injury, post-ictal Worse if pre-existing cognitive deficit	Fluctuating symptoms Drowsiness over hours or days Worse in the afternoon or night Quiet or disruptive Anxiety Agitation	Altered episodes of consciousness Often lucid between episodes Disorientation in time and place Perserveration (word repetition) Delusions Visual hallucinations Impaired short-term memory	
Dementia (See Chronic confusion)				
Personality disorders	Deeply ingrained maladaptive patterns of behaviour The person and/or society suffer Onset only occurs in late teens or early adulthood Determinants of personality: Genetic, neuropsychological, parenting, social mileu (e.g. poverty, culture)	Chronic symptoms Remain unchanged in adult life		May co-exist with anxiety or depression
Subtypes:				
Paranoid personality	Lacking close friends or confidants	Fear of others exploiting or harming them Distrust of friends or associates Sensitive to minor insult	Preoccupied with mistrust/ suspicion	
Schizoid personality	Lacking close friends or confidants	Spend most of their time alone Distant from social relationships Few interests and pleasures in life	Indifferent to praise or criticism Emotionally cold or flat	
Schizotypal personality	Associated with depression May develop transient schizophrenia-like symptoms under stress	Difficulty with close personal relationships Distrust of others	Eccentric Uunusual beliefs in mystical influences that control behaviour Speaks in unusual vague and circumstantial ways No delusions	

Differential Diagnosis in Primary Care, 1st edition. By Nairah Rasul and Mehmood Syed. Published 2009 by Blackwell Publishing, ISBN: 978-1-4051-8036-8

Diagnosis	Background	Key symptoms	Key signs	Additional information
Antisocial personality	Failure to conform to social norms Frequently break the law History of multiple relationships Onset ≤ 15 yrs age M>F Associated with substance abuse Risk of premature violent death	Violate others Little regard for the rights of others Impulsive Irritable Reckless Get into frequent fights	Poor ability to learn from experience No concern for consequences of their actions on themselves or others	
Borderline personality	History of unstable relationships and/or sexual abuse M<F	Intense fear of rejection and loss Rapidly changing moods Feeling of emptiness and boredom	Temporary psychotic episodes Deliberate self-harm Suicidal intent	
Histrionic personality	Dramatic and emotionally labile Risk of deliberate self-harm and substance/alcohol abuse	Crave centre of attention	Excessive display of emotion Attention seeking behaviour Sexually provocative through physical appearance	
Narcissistic personality	Dramatic and emotionally labile M>F Risk of deliberate self-harm and substance/alcohol abuse	Grandiose sense of self-importance Exaggeration of own abilities or achievements Only associate with others perceived as important as themselves	Arrogant attitude Lack of empathy Envious of others Unable to see that others may not appreciate them Preoccupied with fantasies of power and success	
Avoidant personality	History of social inhibition Desires relationships but fearful	Avoids situations whereby criticism may be given Chronic feeling of inadequacy Only involved with new people if sure of praise	Extremely shy and restrained	
Dependent personality	Anxious and fearful	Difficulty making decisions alone Need for others to assume responsibility Difficulty expressing disagreement Difficulty initiating activities due to lack of confidence Fear of disapproval Disproportionate fear of being abandoned Fear of being unable to cope Urgent need to be in a relationship	Seeking constant reassurance	
Obsessive-compulsive personality	Often anxious	Preoccupation with perfectionism, orderliness, control Difficulty with completion of tasks Excessive attention to detail Insist on doing things a certain way Inflexible about money and moral issues Tendency to check and re-check	Lack flexibility or openness Stubborn	

Diagnosis	Background	Key symptoms	Key signs	Additional information
Attention-deficit hyperactive disorder	Children ≤7 yrs age M:F ratio: ≈3:1 Commonly lower social classes Chronic symptoms ≥6 months Present in ≥2 settings (e.g. school, home) Symptoms are maladaptive and inconsistent with developmental level Risk factors: Genetic, learning disorder, family conflict, prenatal exposure to cannabis Associated with: Learning difficulties (e.g. dyslexia), Tourette's, tics, dyspraxia, anxiety	*Inattention:* Forgetfulness Appears not to listen when spoken to Careless mistakes in activities Often fails to complete tasks Difficulty organising tasks/activities Often loses things *Impulsivity:* Lack of social awareness Impatient Often interrupts or intrudes on others *Hyperactivity:* Unable to stay seated Inappropriate running and climbing Often unable to play quietly Constantly on the go	*Inattention:* Easily distracted Poor concentration on tasks *Impulsivity:* Excessive interruption or shouting *Hyperactivity:* Excessive talking Constant fidgeting	Exclude hearing problems
Bipolar affective disorder	Chronic episodic psychotic illness Periods of elation and depression Typical onset in teens and early twenties M<F	Fluctuations in mood From mania or hypomania to depression		Two episodes of severely disturbed mood suggest bipolar One episode must be mania or hypomania
Phases:				
Mania	Severe episode with psychosis	Abnormally elevated mood Overactivity/energetic Disinhibited Impatient and irritable Insomnia Increased appetite for food, drink, sex Reckless expenditure Excessive debt Poor concentration	Bright clothes Psychomotor agitation Pressure of speech Grandiose mood (ambitious) Flight of ideas Sexual disinhibition Heightened perception ± Grandiose delusions ± Persecutory delusions ± Auditory hallucinations ± Lack of insight	Consider hospital admission in severe cases
Hypomania	Mild episode without psychosis Associated with less social dysfunction	Persistent mild elevation of mood Overactivity/energetic	Pressure of speech Flight of ideas No delusions or hallucinations	
Depression		Low mood or anhedonia Lasts most of the day for most days Loss of appetite Weight loss Insomnia Early morning wakening Persistent fatigue Loss of libido Feeling worthless or guilty Poor concentration	Expressionless face Tearful Apathy Uncommunicative Self-neglect Psychomotor retardation Deliberate self-harm Suicidal ideation or intent	Consider hospital admission in severe cases or risk of suicide
Obsessive compulsive disorder	Commonly adolescence and early adulthood M<F Obsessions increase anxiety Compulsions reduce anxiety Risk factors: Depression, anxiety, substance abuse, eating disorder, body dysmorphic disorder Associated with depression	Repetitive bothersome thoughts and actions Unable to get rid of such thoughts Daily activities take longer to complete	*Obsessions:* Involuntary intrusive thoughts *Compulsions:* Physical or mental rituals that have to be completed to control anxiety	

Diagnosis	Background	Key symptoms	Key signs	Additional information
Schizophrenia	Chronic or remitting and relapsing condition Commonest form of psychosis Typical onset late adolescence or early twenties Risk factors: Genetic, intrauterine viral infection, social isolation, migrants, cannabis abuse Positive symptoms may be triggered by acute stress Risk of substance abuse and suicide	*Insidious prodromal phase:* Socially withdrawn Poor attention Low motivation ≥1 *First rank /positive symptoms:* Third-person auditory hallucinations Thought insertion or withdrawal Thought broadcasting Delusions (persecutory or grandiose) External control of emotions Somatic passivity (external control of sensations, thoughts, actions)	Socially withdrawn Suspicious or aggressive Neglect in personal hygiene Disorganised speech Knight's move thinking Use of strange words (neologisms) Incongruent affect Delusions Auditory hallucinations Often lack insight ± Adopt strange uncomfortable postures (catatonia)	Urgent psychiatric assessment Exclude substance abuse and delerium secondary to infection
Autism (Autistic spectrum disorder)	A spectrum of disability Strong genetic predisposition M:F ratio: ≈4:1 Diagnosed from age 18 months ≈70% remain severely handicapped Often require special schooling	*Impaired social communication:* Delayed or absent speech Only talks about a few subjects *Impaired social relationships:* Difficulty forming friendships Little interest in social activities Prefers to be alone *Impaired imagination:* Repetitive play routine Obsession with particular tastes, smells, textures Enjoys a set routine Only tolerates certain foods *Plus:* No response to pain or injury Poor sleep Unprovoked temper tantrums	*Impaired social communication:* Absent "to and fro" conversation Repeats learned phrases inappropriately Poor listening skills Difficulty with abstract concepts (e.g. time) *Impaired social relationships:* Lack of empathy Little or no eye contact Little use or understanding of facial expressions and body language *Impaired imagination:* Repetitive motor movements (e.g. hand flapping, rocking) *Plus:* Unable to follow simple instructions ± Dislike of physical contact	Exclude hearing and sight problems
Asperger's syndrome	Part of autistic spectrum disorder Strong genetic predisposition Causes disruption to daily functioning M:F ratio: ≈4:1 Usually diagnosed from age 2 yrs No linguistic problems IQ normal or above average	Difficulty forming friendships Prefers to be alone Fails to share interests or enjoyment Obsessed with complex subjects Considered "eccentrics" Enjoys a set routine Poor imagination Poor sleep	Normal speech development Normal cognition skills Poor non-verbal skills (e.g. eye contact, facial expression) Unresponsive emotionally or socially Poor motor milestones Repetitive motor movements (e.g. hand flapping and twisting)	
Pre-frontal lobe space occupying lesion	Age >50 yrs Commonly due to a tumour Symptoms develop gradually	New onset headache Worse in morning Progressively worsening Nausea/vomiting Change in personality or behaviour	Drowsiness Cushing's Reflex (BP, HR) Papilloedema (≈50%) Unsteady gait Resistance to passive limb movements (paratonia) Positive unilateral grasp reflex Lack of empathy Disinhibition Reduced social skills	Urgent neurology review
Puerperal psychosis	Risk factors: Personal or family history of psychosis, primiparity High recurrence with subsequent pregnancies	Acute onset 5–15 days postpartum Low mood Emotionally labile Insomnia	Acute confusion Restlessness Anxiety Depression Delusions (may involve infant) Hallucinations Suicidal ideation	Immediate obstetric admission for both mother and child Risk of suicide or harm to the infant

Diagnosis	Background	Key symptoms	Key signs	Additional information
Deliberate self-harm	A non-fatal outcome Usually performed to maintain control in a stressful situation or to cope with a specific problem Commonly teenagers M<F Risk factors: Previous self-harm, depression, anxiety, eating disorder, alcohol/drug abuse, personality disorder, physical abuse, unemployment, criminal record, lower social class, low self-esteem High risk of repeat self-harm and suicide	Deliberate self-harm is impulsive Often in response to acute stress *Common methods:* Self-cutting (e.g. wrists, abdomen) Medication overdose usually with alcohol Ingesting harmful/illicit drugs	Drowsy or LoC Signs of deliberate self-harm ± Depression	Urgent psychiatric assessment to evaluate risk of further harm or suicide 1%–2% risk of completed suicide within 1 yr *Exclude suicidal intent:* A planned act Belief that they would die Did not want to be found Suicidal note An intention to die
Munchausen syndrome	Factitious physical or psychological symptoms Lying about other aspects of life Motivation to adopt the sick role External incentives are absent (e.g. financial) History of numerous investigations and operations	Chronic history of unexplained illness Symptoms are constantly changing Symptoms are vague or detailed A pre-existing condition may be exaggerated or Symptoms simulated or self-induced	Dramatic or hostile behaviour Happy to accept invasive procedures or operations ± Absent or inconsistent clinical signs	May involve factitious symptoms in another child or adult (Munchausen's by proxy)

Anxiety

Diagnosis	Background	Key symptoms	Key signs	Additional information
Panic disorder	History of discrete episodes of anxiety (panic attacks) Intense subjective fear with symptomatic manifestations Unanticipated attacks Variable in frequency Attack lasts <1 h Chronic anxiety >1 month Anxiety related to subsequent attacks or effects of attack Agoraphobia may co-exist ≈50% develop depression	Fast palpitations Chest discomfort/pain Shortness of breath Dizziness Nausea/vomiting Numbness and tingling "Fear of losing control"	No physical signs between attacks *During an attack:* Hyperventilation Sweating Sinus tachycardia Hypertension Severe anxiety Affect congruent with mental state Fear of death/illness ± Suicidal ideation	Exclude alcohol/drug misuse
Generalised anxiety disorder	Usually chronic persistent anxiety Excessive or unrealistic worry Inappropriate to the situation Affects daily functioning Associated with stress and depression	Fast palpitations Shortness of breath Dizziness Nausea/vomiting Numbness and tingling "Fear of losing control" Poor concentration Insomnia Urinary frequency Frequent or loose bowel motions Erectile dysfunction	Hyperventilation Sweating Sinus tachycardia Hypertension Severe anxiety Fear of death/illness Postural hand tremor	Exclude alcohol/drug misuse
Post-traumatic stress disorder	History of a recent threatening or catastrophic event Involves oneself or others Recurrent and chronic symptoms High-risk groups: Elderly, children, veterans, mental health patients, refugees	Recurrent flashbacks of the event Diffiulty falling or staying asleep Nightmares Avoidance of situations likely to trigger memories Loss of interest in other activities Jumpy and easily startled Increased vigilance Low mood Poor concentration Loss of libido	Constant fear and anxiety Depression ± Drug and/or alcohol abuse	Risk of: Alcohol and drug abuse, somatisation, chronic pain, poor health

Diagnosis	Background	Key symptoms	Key signs	Additional information
Obsessive compulsive disorder	Commonly adolescence and early adulthood M<F Obsessions increase anxiety Compulsions reduce anxiety Risk factors: Depression, anxiety, substance abuse, eating disorder, body dysmorphic disorder Associated with depression	Repetitive bothersome thoughts and actions Unable to get rid of such thoughts Daily activities take longer to complete	*Obsessions:* Involuntary intrusive thoughts *Compulsions:* Physical or mental rituals that have to be completed out to control anxiety	
Phobias	A strong fear or dread of a thing or event Disproportionate to the situation Considered disruptive to one's life	Anxiety is not constant Only occurs in certain circumstances *Plus physical symptoms:* Sweating Palpitations Dry mouth Nausea Shaking Avoidance of feared situation Anticipation of situation leads to anxiety	Disproportionate level of anxiety	
Hypochondriasis	A subtype of somatisation Usually secondary to illness or personality disorder Commonly middle-aged or elderly M>F History of repeated investigations	Preoccupation with physical ill health and bodily sensations Fear of having a serious disease despite reassurance Symptoms are often non-specific (e.g. diffuse pain) Symptoms not intentionally produced	Increasing anxiety Disproportionate to any existing physical disorder Profound belief in being sick Seeking constant reassurance	

Low mood

Diagnosis	Background	Key symptoms	Key signs	Additional information
Depression	Risk factors: Genetic, lower social class Precipitating factors include: Bereavement, job loss, relationship break-up, chronic illness, drugs (e.g. beta-blockers), pregnancy Can be part of a bipolar disorder	Low mood or anhedonia Lasts most of the day for most days Loss of appetite Weight loss Insomnia Early morning awakening Persistent fatigue Loss of libido Feeling worthless or guilty Poor concentration	Expressionless face Tearful Apathy Uncommunicative Self-neglect Psychomotor retardation Deliberate self-harm Suicidal ideation or intent	Consider hospital admission in severe cases or risk of suicide
Postnatal depression				
Subtypes:				
Maternity/Baby blues	Risk factors: First pregnancy, depression in last trimester, previous history of PMT Resolves within hours to a few days with support and reassurance	Onset 3–6 days postpartum Labile mood Tearful Irritable Anxious about coping Fatigue	No depression No psychosis	

Diagnosis	Background	Key symptoms	Key signs	Additional information
Depressive illness	Non-psychotic depression Onset within 1 yr postpartum Commonly within 3 to 6 months Affects mother-to-infant bonding Common risk factors: Previous depression, lack of social support, marital conflict, recent adverse life events	Gradual onset low mood Onset ≥2 wks postpartum Tearful Irritable Loss of enjoyment in having baby Inability to cope Feeling hopeless Low self-esteem Poor sleep Poor appetite Poor concentration Low energy levels Loss of libido	Moderate to severe depression No psychosis	Exclude hypothyroidism Avoid progesterone-only contraceptives Immediate referral if risk of suicide, self-harm or harm to infant
Puerperal psychosis	Risk factors: Personal or family history of psychosis, primiparity High recurrence with subsequent pregnancies	Acute onset 5–15 days postpartum Low mood Emotionally labile Insomnia	Acute confusion Restlessness Anxiety Depression Delusions (may involve infant) Hallucinations Suicidal ideation	Immediate obstetric admission for both mother and child Beware risk of suicide or harm to the infant
Dementia (See Chronic confusion)				
Acute drug or alcohol intoxication (See Dizziness)				
Post-traumatic stress disorder	History of a recent threatening or catastrophic event Involves oneself or others Recurrent and chronic symptoms High-risk groups: Elderly, children, veterans, mental health patients, refugees	Recurrent flashbacks of the event Difficulty falling or staying asleep Nightmares Avoidance of situations likely to trigger memories Loss of interest in other activities Jumpy and easily startled Increased vigilance Low mood Poor concentration Loss of libido	Constant fear and anxiety Depression ± Drug and/or alcohol abuse	Risk of: Alcohol and drug abuse, somatisation, chronic pain, poor health
Seasonal affective disorder	A type of depression Related to seasonal variations in daylight Seasonal symptoms present for ≥2 consecutive years Commonly ≈30 yrs age M<F Associated with eating disorders	Low mood for most of the day Over-eating Weight gain Over-sleeping Poor concentration Symptoms worse during autumn/winter Relieved in spring/summer	Often atypical signs of depression	Exclude self-harm or suicidal ideation
Acquired hypothyroidism	Age >60 yrs M<F Causes: Autoimmune, thyroiditis, TSH deficiency, postpartum, thyroidectomy, neck radiation, iodine deficiency, drugs (e.g. amiodarone, carbizamole) Associated with high cholesterol/triglycerides and anaemia	Lethargy Weight gain Low mood Cold intolerance Menorrhagia	Deep hoarse voice Slow cognition (e.g. poor memory) Dry coarse skin Thinning of hair Bradycardia Slow-relaxing tendon reflexes ± Goitre	Beware myxoedema in the elderly: Puffy eyes, hands and feet Cerebellar ataxia Hypothermia Seizures ± Coma
Bipolar affective disorder (See Abnormal behaviour)				

Chapter 12
Miscellaneous

Acute confusion

Diagnosis	Background	Key symptoms	Key signs	Additional information
Alcohol intoxication	Common in teenagers and young adults	History of alcohol abuse	Smell of alcohol Slurred speech Incoordination Unsteady gait Nystagmus Facial flushing Aggressive or disinhibited behaviour	Beware of co-existing head injury or hypoglycaemia as a true cause of confusion
Infection	Common causes: UTI, pneumonia, sepsis, meningitis	Malaise Anorexia Nausea/vomiting	Fever Tachycardia Tachypnoea Other signs according to underlying cause	
Hypoxia	Commonly due to respiratory or cardiac failure History of lung and/or heart disease	Shortness of breath Reduced exercise tolerance	Central cyanosis Tachypnoea Tachycardia ± Pulmonary oedema ± Peripheral oedema	May be precipitated by underlying infection (e.g. pneumonia)
Hypoglycaemia	Possible history of pre-existing or undiagnosed DM Causes: Insulin/oral hypoglycaemics, sulfonylurea, alcohol binge, pituitary insufficiency, liver failure, Addison's disease, insulinoma, post gastric surgery	Lethargy Sweating Hunger Tremor Paraesthesia of lips and tongue Poor concentration	Apyrexial No cyanosis Finger-prick blood glucose <3.0 mmol/litre Slurred speech ± Transient hemiplegia (rarely in IDDM) ± LoC	
Hyponatraemia	Causes of dehydration: Addison's disease, renal failure, diuretics, diarrhoea, vomiting, fistula, burns, small bowel obstruction, CF, heat stroke Causes of oedema: Nephrotic syndrome, cardiac failure, cirrhosis, renal failure Other causes: Inappropriate ADH secretion, water overload, severe hypothyroidism	Depend on level and rate of sodium decline *Common symptoms:* Anorexia Nausea/vomiting Lethargy Muscle cramps and weakness Acute confusion Drowsiness (in severe cases)	Depend on level and rate of sodium decline *Dehydration:* Tachycardia Dry mucous membranes Diminshed skin turgor Or *fluid overload:* Peripheral oedema Ascites Raised JVP	Beware pseudohyponatraemia due to high serum lipids/proteins or hyperglycaemia
Hypernatraemia	Causes include: Excess fluid loss, excess i.v. saline, diabetes insipidus, primary hyperaldosteronism, renal failure At-risk groups: Elderly, infirm, infants with diarrhoea and inadequate milk feeding	Acute confusion Thirst Lethargy Irritable Tremor Oliguria ± Seizures	Drowsy Dehydration Hyper-reflexia ± Postural hypotension ± Tachycardia	Rapid rehydration can cause cerebral oedema

Differential Diagnosis in Primary Care, 1st edition. By Nairah Rasul and Mehmood Syed. Published 2009 by Blackwell Publishing, ISBN: 978-1-4051-8036-8

Diagnosis	Background	Key symptoms	Key signs	Additional information
Hypercalcaemia	Common causes: Primary hyperparathyroidism, malignancy, CRF Risk of cardiac arrhythmia due to shortened QT interval	Vary depending on severity *Common symptoms:* Upper abdominal pain Lethargy Low mood Polyuria Polydipsia Constipation Muscle weakness	Acute confusion Dehydration	Long-term complications include renal stones and chondrocalcinosis Avoid thiazides
Silent myocardial infarction	Commonly elderly or diabetic Risk factors: Advancing age, male gender, family history, South Asian, obesity, hyperlipidaemia, DM, smoking, hypertension	Malaise No chest pain	Low-grade fever <39°C Anxiety Cold and clammy Systolic murmur ± Heart failure ± LoC	Emergency admission
Cerebrovascular accident (See Dysphagia)				
Diabetic ketoacidosis	Hyperglycaemia and ketoacidosis Often due to Type I DM Develops over hours/days Commonly young adults Risk factors: Infection, inadequate insulin, new onset DM, MI, CVA, pregnancy, alcohol abuse, new medication (e.g. steroids, beta blockers)	Polyuria Polydipsia Nausea/vomiting Weight loss Non-specific abdominal pain	Severe dehydration Ketotic breath Tachypnoea Tachycardia ± Acute confusion ± Infection (e.g. URTI, UTI) *Abnormal urinalysis:* Glycosuria ± Ketonuria	
Post-ictal state	History of recent seizure Collateral history useful Provoking factors: Fever, brain trauma or infection, hypoglycaemia, electrolyte abnormality, CVA, alcohol excess, drug withdrawal, drugs (e.g. theophylline)	Symptoms last hours to 2 days Lethargy Poor concentration Poor short-term memory Drowsy Migraine Low mood	Reduced level of consciousness Confusion	Consider referral in unprovoked seizures (For Epilepsy, see Syncope)
Delirium tremens	Autonomic dysfunction Due to chronic alcohol abuse followed by acute withdrawal Risk factors for alcohol abuse: Previous history, family history, binge drinking, poverty, emotional stress, drug addiction, occupation (e.g. publican) Associated with social and mental health problems	Onset symptoms ≤1 wk from cessation or reduction in alcohol Apprehension Agitation Worse at night	Fever Hypertension Tachycardia Dilated pupils Sweating Disorientation in time and place Reduced level of consciousness Coarse hand tremor Impaired short-term memory Hallucinations (tactile and visual) ± Seizures ± Cirrhosis	Emergency medical admission
Drug and substance abuse	May involve overdosage of prescribed medication Common in the elderly Common drugs: Narcotic analgesics, benzodiazepines, warfarin, frusemide, captopril, TCA, dipyridamole, theophylline, beta-blockers, digoxin, steroids	History of polypharmacy ± Dementia	Signs vary depending on medication	
Other commonly abused drugs:				
Glue or solvent abuse	Common inhalants: Cleaning solvents, hydrofluorocarbon aerosols, glue, nail polish removers, fuels Commonly teenagers or people who do not have access to other drugs	Acute onset symptoms Agitation Headache Nausea/vomiting	Smell of solvents Perioral or nasal rash Euphoria Confusion Hallucinations Slurred speech Unsteady gait	High risk of death from aspiration of vomit and hypoxia

Diagnosis	Background	Key symptoms	Key signs	Additional information
CNS depressants	Common CNS depressants: Barbiturates, benzodiazepines, alcohol, narcotics, antihistamines, ketamines Possible history of insomnia and anxiety	Dizziness Drowsy Feeling calm	Reduced level of consciousness Nystagmus Moderately dilated pupils Diplopia Strabismus Hypotonia Loss in coordination ± Injection scars	Abrupt withdrawal of long-term benzodiazepines can have serious side-effects
Amphetamines and cocaine	Associated with higher social classes	Chest pain (may indicate MI) Restlessness	Fever Malignant hyperthermia Hyperstimulation Widely dilated pupils Paranoid behaviour Violent behaviour Cardiac arrhythmias	
Head injury	Extradural haemorrhage Due to fractured temporal or parietal bone Laceration of middle meningeal artery and/or vein	History of recent head trauma Initially no LoC post-injury Any drowsiness resolves temporarily *Hours to days post-trauma:* Drowsiness Severe headache Vomiting ± Seizures	Confusion Altered level of consciousness Hemiparesis Brisk reflexes Upgoing plantars *Severe signs:* Coma Ipsilateral pupil dilatation Deep and irregular breathing Bilateral spastic paraparesis	Emergency CT head
Hyperthyroid crisis (Thyrotoxic storm)	Severe hyperthyroidism Often history of Graves' disease Risk factors: Recent thyroid surgery or radioiodine, infection, MI, DKA, hypoglycaemia, trauma (e.g. surgery), deficient anti-thyroid medication	Agitation Diarrhoea Vomiting Abdominal pain	High-grade fever >39°C Dehydration Jaundice Hypotension Tachycardia Acute confusion or coma Goitre Thyroid bruit ± Atrial fibrillation	
Wernicke's encephalopathy	Thiamine (Vitamin B1) deficiency Involved in transketolase enzyme function Risk factors: Chronic alcohol abuse, malnutrition, eating disorders, prolonged vomiting	Anorexia Headache Unsteady gait	Ataxic gait Acute confusion Mild memory impairment Reduced level of consciousness Hypothermia Hypotension Oculomotor problems: Nystagmus Irregular pupil size Bilateral lateral rectus palsy	If untreated, progresses to memory problems and confabulation (Korsakoff syndrome)

Chronic confusion

Diagnosis	Background	Key symptoms	Key signs	Additional information
Dementia	Middle-aged and elderly Global impairment of intellect, memory and personality	Gradual onset over months/years Progressive deterioration over time	No drowsiness	Exclude treatable causes: B12/folate/thyroid deficiency Syphilis Depression Cerebral mass
Common subtypes:				
Alzheimer's disease	Age >40 yrs M<F Often sporadic May be familial Risk factors: Advancing age, Caucasian	Insidious onset cognitive decline Symptoms occur all day Interference with daily living *Late symptoms:* Aggression Mutism Wandering or immobility Incontinence Delusions and hallucinations	Memory impairment *Plus ≥1 of the following:* Agnosia Aphasia (spoken or written) Apraxia Difficulty in organising and planning Normal neurological examination Mini-mental test ≤23/30	

Diagnosis	Background	Key symptoms	Key signs	Additional information
Multi-infarct (Vascular)	History of repeat small CVAs Risk factors: Atherosclerosis, hypertension	Symptoms may be acute Stepwise decline in cognition Symptom severity varies in the day Usually worse in the evening	Small steps on walking (marche a petit pas) Parkinsonism *Spasticity:* Increased limb tone Resistance to passive movement Hyperreflexia	
Lewy body dementia	Lewy body: neuronal inclusion body throughout the cortex	Fluctuating confusion	Recurrent visual hallucinations Delusions Impaired visuospatial skills *Mild spontaneous parkinsonism:* Bradykinesia Festinated gait Resting "pill rolling" hand tremor Cogwheel rigidity Expressionless face	
Cerebral tumour	History of malignancy May be primary or secondary Gliomas are the commonest primary brain tumour in adults	Gradual onset symptoms Generalised headache Worse in the morning Aggravated by stooping Vomiting Progressive confusion Visual disturbances Personality changes Seizures	Unsteady gait Reduced level of consciousness Falling pulse and rising BP (Cushing's reflex) Focal neurology Papilloedema	
Liver failure	Fulminant (<8 wks) or late-onset (>8 wks) liver failure Common causes: Paracetamol overdose, viral infection, drug toxicity, cirrhosis, hepatocarcinoma, autoimmune, Budd-Chiari syndrome, acute fatty liver of pregnancy	*Grade I encephalopathy:* Mild confusion Altered mood or behaviour *Grade II encephalopathy:* Progressive confusion Drowsiness Difficulty performing mental tasks Slurred speech *Grade III encephalopathy:* Somnolent but rousable Incomprehensible speech *Grade IV encephalopathy:* Coma	Jaundice Ascites Palmar erythema Flapping tremor (encephalopathy) ± Hepatosplenomegaly	Complications include: Sepsis, GI bleeding, cerebral oedema, renal failure, respiratory failure
Huntingdon's chorea	Progressive neurodegenerative movement disorder Autosomal dominant Abnormal gene on chromosome 4 Typical onset middle-age	Early personality changes Seizures Dysphagia Irritability Self-neglect	Progressive dementia Dysarthria Chorea (rapid involuntary jerks) Dystonia (repetitive twisting movements and abnormal posture) *Late signs:* Clonus Spasticity Upgoing plantars	
Creutzfeldt-Jakob disease	Due to human CNS infection with prion protein Commonly sporadic Other causes: Iatrogenic, familial, new variant prion New variant prion (nvCJD) linked to eating infected meats with BSE	Symptoms are rapidly progressive Behavioural changes Anxiety Low mood	Cerebellar ataxia Dementia Myoclonic jerks Focal neurology	Prognosis of fatal illness varies: Sporadic CJD may be fatal within a few months Familial and nvCJD often survive >1 yr

Dizziness (lightheadedness)

Diagnosis	Background	Key symptoms	Key signs	Additional information
Viral illness	Usually self-limiting Droplet spread	Gradual onset dizziness Persistent No illusion of movement Lethargy	Normal gait No postural drop Normal heart sounds	
Generalised anxiety disorder	Usually chronic and persistent anxiety Excessive or unrealistic worry Inappropriate to the situation Affects daily functioning Associated with stress and depression	Fast palpitations Shortness of breath Dizziness Nausea/vomiting Numbness and tingling "Fear of losing control" Poor concentration Insomnia Urinary frequency Frequent or loose bowel motions Erectile dysfunction	Hyperventilation Sweating Sinus tachycardia Hypertension Severe anxiety Fear of death/illness Postural hand tremor	Exclude alcohol/drug misuse
Postural hypotension (Orthostatic hypotension)	Transient impaired cerebral perfusion Commonly elderly Causes: Medication, prolonged standing, prolonged bedrest, hypovolaemia, diabetic autonomic neuropathy, Addison's disease, idiopathic	Acute onset dizziness or syncope Worse on standing Relieved by lying down No illusion of movement ± Falls with no LoC	Postural drop >20 mmHg systolic on standing Unsteady on abrupt standing Normal heart sounds	
Hypoglycaemia (See Acute confusion)				
Acute drug or alcohol intoxication	Alcohol or illicit drug abuse	Recent drug or excess alcohol intake Acute onset dizziness Falls ± LoC ± Vomiting ± Labile mood (e.g. low mood)	Dehydration Unsteady gait Unable to walk heel to toe ± Slurred speech ± Hallucinations	
Post-concussion syndrome (See Headache)				
Aortic stenosis	Causes: Senile calcification, congenital Results in LVH This can progress to CCF Associated with bacterial endocarditis and sudden death	*Symptoms occur on exertion:* Breathlessness Angina ± Dizziness or syncope	Slow rising pulse Small volume pulse Narrow pulse pressure Palpable LV heave Palpable systolic thrill Soft or absent S2 Ejection systolic murmur Loudest at aortic area and left sternal edge Radiates to apex and carotids	Aortic sclerosis sounds similar but is distinguished from aortic stenosis by: Normal pulse Normal S2 No radiation to carotids Absent systolic thrill
Carbon monoxide poisoning	Risk of fits and coma in prolonged exposure	Nausea/vomiting Dizziness Worse when heater or cooking appliance in use Relieved when away from house	Pink skin and oral mucosa Tachypnoea Tachycardia	Check gas appliances and flues

Falls with no loss of consciousness

Diagnosis	Background	Key symptoms	Key signs	Additional information
Postural instability	Commonly age >65 yrs Increase prevalance with age Risk factors: Muscle weakness, limited mobility (e.g. OA), assisted device (e.g. walking stick)	Able to recall the events of the fall No symptoms prior to fall	Muscle wasting (e.g. quadriceps) Normal sensation intact No confusion No postural drop in BP	Exclude impaired vision Consider home safety assessment to rule out trip hazards (e.g. loose rugs, poor lighting)
Postural hypotension (Orthostatic hypotension)	Transient impaired cerebral perfusion Commonly elderly Causes: Medication, prolonged standing, prolonged bedrest, hypovolaemia, diabetic autonomic neuropathy, Addison's disease, idiopathic	Acute onset dizziness or syncope Worse on standing Relieved by lying down No illusion of movement	Postural drop >20 mmHg systolic on standing Unsteady on abrupt standing Normal heart sounds	
CVA or TIA (See Dysphagia)				
Vertigo (See Ear, nose and throat)				
Medication	Associated with polypharmacy Common drugs: Antihypertensives, benzodiazapines, antipsychotics, antidepressants, anticonvulsants	History of falls after taking medication ± Drowsiness	Normal heart sounds ± Postural drop ± Confusion	
Acute drug or alcohol intoxication	Alcohol or illicit drug abuse	Recent drug or excess alcohol intake Acute onset dizziness Falls ± LoC ± Vomiting ± Labile mood	Dehydration Unsteady gait Unable to walk heel to toe ± Slurred speech ± Hallucinations	
Parkinson's disease	Idiopathic movement disorder Degeneration of substantia nigra dopaminergic neurones Degenerating neurones contain Lewy bodies Peak onset 55–65 yrs age Other causes of parkinsonism: Drug-induced (e.g. neuroleptics), post-encephalitis, toxins, head trauma, Wilson's disease, Lewy body dementia, vascular dementia	Recurrent falls with no LoC Resting hand tremor Worse with stress Relieved by voluntary movement Dysphagia and dribbling Low mood in ≈50%	Festinated (shuffling steps) gait Unilateral resting "pill rolling" tremor Generalised tremor years later Bradykinesia Expressionless face Monotonous speech Cogwheel or lead-pipe rigidity during passive limb movement Present in flexors and extensors Micrographia Normal muscle power Normal tendon reflexes Normal plantar responses	Late onset dementia may develop after ≈10 yrs
Cardiac arrhythmia (See Heart murmurs)				

Fatigue

Diagnosis	Background	Key symptoms	Key signs	Additional information
Insomnia (See Insomnia)				
Diabetes mellitus	Predisposing factors for DKA or HONK: Any infection, inadequate insulin or non-compliance, undiagnosed DM, illness (e.g. MI, CVA), drugs (e.g. beta-blockers, diuretics)			Inform DVLA Complications: CVA, MI, retinopathy, limb ischaemia, neuropathy, infections
Subtypes:				
Type I diabetes	Lack of endogenous insulin Commonly children or young adults Associated with autoimmune disease Risk of ketoacidosis Presentation is acute or subacute Longer history of symptoms	*Acute diabetic ketoacidosis:* Acute onset symptoms Fatigue Malaise Weight loss Polyuria and frequency Polydipsia Nausea/vomiting Non-specific abdominal pain *Subacute symptoms:* Fatigue Weight loss Polyuria and frequency Polydipsia Plus recurrent infections (e.g. boils, thrush, UTI)	*Acute diabetic ketoacidosis:* Severe dehydration Tachycardia Tachypnoea Ketotic breath ± Confusion ± Infection (e.g. URTI, UTI) *Abnormal urinalysis:* Glucose Ketones *Subacute signs:* *Abnormal urinalysis:* Glucose ± Ketones	DKA warrants emergency admission
Type II diabetes	Reduced insulin secretion Increased insulin resistance Typical age >40 yrs Commonest type of diabetes Common risk factors: Obesity, South Asian, Afro-Caribbean, male gender, family history, gestational DM, impaired glucose tolerance, metabolic syndrome, drugs (e.g. steroids) Not prone to ketoacidosis Presents insidiously or subacutely with HONK	*Insidious onset:* Weight loss Polyuria and frequency Polydipsia *Hyperosmolar non-ketotic coma:* Gradual onset symptoms over ≥1 wk Generalised weakness Lethargy ± Seizures	*Insidious onset:* Few signs may be present Glycosuria *Hyperosmolar non-ketotic coma:* Severe dehydration Tachycardia Confusion Reduced level of consciousness Finger-prick glucose >30 mmol/litre ± Focal CNS signs (e.g. hemiparesis) ± Infection *Abnormal urinalyis:* Glucose No ketones	May eventually require insulin HONK warrants emergency admission High risk of DVT
Depression (See Low mood)				
Acquired hypothyroidism	Age >60 yrs M<F Causes: Autoimmune, thyroiditis, TSH deficiency, postpartum, thyroidectomy, neck radiation, iodine deficiency, drugs (e.g. amiodarone, carbizamole) Associated with high cholesterol/triglycerides and anaemia	Lethargy Weight gain Low mood Cold intolerance Menorrhagia	Deep hoarse voice Slow cognition (e.g. poor memory) Dry coarse skin Thinning of hair Bradycardia Slow-relaxing tendon reflexes ± Goitre	Beware myxoedema in the elderly: Puffy eyes, hands and feet Cerebellar ataxia Hypothermia Seizures ± Coma
Anaemia (See Chronic breathlessness)				
Medication	Common drugs: Cytotoxic, beta-blockers, tranquilisers, antidepressants	Onset of fatigue after taking medication	Vary according to medication taken	

Diagnosis	Background	Key symptoms	Key signs	Additional information
Obstructive sleep apnoea	Intermittent upper airway collapse Occurs during sleep Results in irregular breathing Relieved by partial arousal Typically middle-aged M>F Risk factors: Obesity, smoking, sedative drugs, excess alcohol	Loud snoring Choking episodes during sleep Unrefreshing sleep Daytime fatigue and somnolence Poor concentration Irritable Reduced libido ± Witnessed apnoeic episodes	Often normal ENT examination ± BMI ≥30 kg/m² ± Neck circumference >17 inches ± Craniofacial or pharyngeal abnormalities (e.g. micrognathia, enlarged tonsils)	Complications: PHT, Type II respiratory failure, hypertension, CCF
Chronic fatigue syndrome (Myalgic encephalomyelitis)	Commonly age ≥30 yrs M:F ratio: ≈1:2 A diagnosis of exclusion Chronic symptoms >3 months Wide range of symptoms Worse after physical or mental exertion Associated with depression	Persistent or recurrent fatigue Worse after exertion Not relieved by rest Post-exertional malaise Typically delayed >24 h after exertion Usually lasts a few days Reduced ADL *Plus ≥1 of the following:* Disturbed sleep pattern Multiple arthralgia Multiple myalgia Headaches Sore throat Cognitive dysfunction (e.g .poor concentration) Generalised malaise Painful LN	Unremarkable examination Tender LN without swelling No joint swelling	
Fibromyalgia	Age 25–55 yrs M:F ratio: ≈1:7	Generalised body pain Insomnia Chronic fatigue Low mood Anxiety	Systemically well Depression Pain over specific trigger points No red flag signs No arthralgia	Red flag signs: Age <20 yrs or >55 yrs Abnormal neurology Thoracic back pain Weight loss Fever History of malignancy Use of systemic steroids
Multiple sclerosis	Chronic condition Autoimmune demyelinating disorder Affects CNS only Commonly young adults M:F ratio: ≈2:3 Commonest cause of neurological disability in the young	Blurred vision Visual loss Double vision Urgency Impotence Leg weakness Numbness of perineum and genitalia Bowel and/or bladder incontinence Paraesthesia of limbs Vertigo Incoordination	*Focal neurological deficit:* Symmetrical horizontal nystagmus Optic neuritis Cranial nerve lesions Cerebellar signs *UMN limb weakness:* No muscle wasting Spasticity Hypertonia Brisk reflexes Upgoing plantar response	
Polymyalgia rheumatica	Inflammatory conditon Affects shoulder and pelvic girdle Age >50 yrs M:F ratio: ≈1:3	Pain around shoulders and pelvis Morning stiffness Difficulty getting out of bed Weight loss Joint swelling	Fever Pain on active and passive movement of shoulders, neck, hips Muscle tenderness	Giant cell arteritis may co-exist
Leukaemia (See Petechiae and ecchymoses)				
Adenoid hyperplasia	Pre-pubescent children Adenoids normally atrophy by age ≤15 yrs Associated with recurrent middle ear infection/effusion and sinusitis	Mouth breathing often at night Daytime fatigue (due to lack of sleep) Otalgia Deafness ± Sleep apnoea	Evidence of recurrent URTI ± Enlarged tonsils	Persitent fatigue can cause problems at school Consider ENT referral

Heart murmurs

Diagnosis	Background	Key symptoms	Key signs	Additional information
Aortic stenosis	Causes: Senile calcification, congenital Results in LVH This can progress to CCF Associated with bacterial endocarditis and sudden death	*Symptoms worse on exertion:* Shortness of breath Angina ± Dizziness or syncope	Slow rising pulse Small volume pulse Narrow pulse pressure Palpable LV heave Palpable systolic thrill Soft or absent S2 Ejection systolic murmur Loudest at aortic area and left sternal edge Radiates to apex and carotids	Aortic sclerosis sounds similar but is distinguished from aortic stenosis by: Normal pulse Normal S2 No radiation to carotids Absent systolic thrill
Aortic regurgitation (Aortic incompetence)	Cusp abormality or aortic root dilatation Causes of cusp abnormality: Congenital, rheumatic fever, endocarditis Causes of root dilatation: Idiopathic, hypertension, seronegative arthritides (e.g. ankylosing spondylitis), aortic dissection, Marfan's syndrome Results mainly in LV dilatation This can progress to LVF	Typically asymptomatic or Shortness of breath (in LVF) Palpitations	Collapsing ("waterhammer") pulse Wide pulse pressure Displaced apex Early high-pitched diastolic murmur Loudest at aortic area and apex Heard best in expiration on sitting forward Corrigan's sign (carotid pulsation)	
Mitral regurgitation (Mitral incompetence)	Acute or chronic Primary or secondary Common primary causes: Valve prolapse, annular calcification, rheumatic fever, inferior MI, connective tissue disorder (e.g. Marfan's syndrome), congenital Secondary causes due to chronic LV dilatation (e.g. dilated cardiomyopathy) Results in dilated LA and LV	Fatigue Shortness of breath Palpitations	Atrial fibrillation (in dilated LA) RV and LV heave Displaced apex Soft or reduced S1 Soft pansystolic murmur Loudest at apex Radiates to axilla ± Split S2 and loud P2 (in pulmonary hypertension)	Complications: LVF, ventricular ectopics, infective endocarditis
Mitral stenosis	Commonly due to rheumatic fever M<F Results in dilated LA Associated with progressive right axis deviation	Fatigue Shortness of breath Palpitations Chest pain Haemoptysis	Malar flush Low volume pulse AF Tapping undisplaced apex Loud S1 ± Loud P2 ± Followed by early mitral opening snap Rumbling mid-diastolic murmur Loudest at apex Heard best in expiration when lying on left side Pulmonary oedema	Complications: PHT, RHF, atrial thromboembolism
Pulmonary stenosis	Commonly congenital: Turner's syndrome, Fallot's tetralogy Acquired causes: Carcinoid syndrome, rheumatic fever Results in dilated right atrium and ventricle Associated with right axis deviation, RBBB, RVH	Fatigue Breathless on exertion Leg and abdominal swelling Nausea Anorexia	Normal pulse Left parasternal RV heave Ejection sytolic murmur Loudest at upper left sternal edge Radiates to left clavicle and beneath left scapula ± Split S2 (delayed P2) *Right ventricular failure:* Raised JVP (large A wave) Leg and sacral pitting oedema Ascites Hepatomegaly (may be pulsatile) ± Mild jaundice ± Cyanosis	

Diagnosis	Background	Key symptoms	Key signs	Additional information
Tricuspid regurgitation	Causes: RVF, endocarditis (i.v. drug abusers), rheumatic fever, congenital, carcinoid syndrome Results in dilated right atrium and ventricle Associated with RVH or RBBB	Fatigue Shortness of breath Hepatic pain on exertion Leg and abdominal swelling	Left parasternal RV heave Pansystolic murmur Loudest at lower left sternal edge Best heard in inspiration ± AF *Right ventricular failure:* Jaundice Raised JVP Leg and sacral pitting oedema Ascites Pulsatile hepatomegaly	
Atrial septal defect	Commonly ostium secundum A persistent foetal foramen ovale (high septal defect) Results in left to right atrial shunt Can lead to PHT and pulmonary or tricuspid regurgitation Associated with: RAD, RVH, RBBB Spontaneous closure may occur	Typical onset in early adulthood Breathless on exertion Recurrent chest infections	Late onset AF Raised JVP Left parasternal RV heave Loud ejection systolic murmur Loudest over left 2nd intercostal space Wide fixed split S2 in respiration	Complications include reversal of left to right shunt (Eisenmenger syndrome)
Ventricular septal defect	Congenital (Down's syndrome, rubella) or acquired (post-MI, trauma) Smaller defects are associated with a louder murmur ≈60% of small defects close spontaneously	Asymptomatic if small defect or Shortness of breath Recurrent chest infections Failure to thrive	Normal pulse Normal JVP Harsh pansystolic murmur Loudest at left lower sternal edge Radiates all over pericardium Palpable systolic thrill ± Left parasternal RV heave	Complications: Aortic regurgitation, endocarditis, PHT, Eisenmenger syndrome
Patent ductus arteriosus	Congenital Blood flow from aorta to pulmonary artery Usually closes within 48 h of life Can take up to 3 months if preterm M<F Risk factors: Congenital rubella, prematurity Results in left ventricular fluid overload Associated with LVH	Often asymptomatic or Fatigue Failure to thrive Breathless on exertion Reccurent chest infections	Large volume pulse Normal JVP Prominent apex beat Loud continuous "machinery" murmur Loudest under left clavicle	Complications include: PHT and cardiac failure
Coarctation of the aorta	Aortic narrowing at or distal to origin of left subclavian artery M>F Associated with: Turner's syndrome, gestational DM, congenital heart defects (e.g. VSD)	Symptoms often occur after many years Headaches due to high BP Claudication	Hypertension Radiofemoral delay or Absent femoral pulses Mid to late systolic murmur Cold legs	Can cause early cardiac failure in neonates

Insomnia

Diagnosis	Background	Key symptoms	Key signs	Additional information
Acute stress	Recent stressful life event: Exams, new job, divorce, redundancy, bereavement, moving house Usually resolves with time	History of recent stressful event Reduced appetite Mild anxiety Normal mood	Systemically well No depression	
Poor sleep hygiene	Commonly elderly M<F Common causes: Excess caffeine or alcohol, nicotine, drugs, TV, disturbed sleep routine (e.g.shift work, jet-lag), daytime naps, exercise Shift workers have a higher risk of depression	Difficulty falling asleep No early morning awakening No weight loss Normal mood ± Anxiety about not getting to sleep	Systemically well	Sleep requirements tend to fall with increasing age Avoid prescribing hypnotics in the elderly due to risk of falls from confusion and drowsiness Beware of drug addicts trying to obtain benzodiazapines

Diagnosis	Background	Key symptoms	Key signs	Additional information
Generalised anxiety disorder	Usually chronic and persistent anxiety Excessive or unrealistic worry Inappropriate to the situation Affects daily functioning Associated with stress and depression	Fast palpitations Shortness of breath Dizziness Nausea/vomiting Numbness and tingling "Fear of losing control" Poor concentration Insomnia Urinary frequency Frequent or loose bowel motions Erectile dysfunction	Hyperventilation Sweating Sinus tachycardia Hypertension Severe anxiety Fear of death/illness Postural hand tremor	Exclude alcohol/drug misuse
Depression	Risk factors: Genetic, lower social class Precipitating factors include: Bereavement, job loss, relationship break-up, chronic illness, drugs (e.g. beta-blockers), pregnancy Can be part of a bipolar disorder	Low mood or anhedonia Lasts most of the day for most days Loss of appetite Weight loss Insomnia Early morning awakening Reduced energy or fatigue Loss of libido Feeling worthless or guilty Poor concentration	Expressionless face Tearful Apathy Uncommunicative Self-neglect Psychomotor retardation Deliberate self-harm Suicidal ideation or intent	Consider hospital admission in severe cases or risk of suicide
Chronic pain	Common causes: Arthritis, headache, backache, cramps	Difficulty falling or staying asleep Intermittent awakening by pain ± Low mood	Vary depending on underlying cause	New onset bony pain that disturbs sleep requires further investigation to exclude malignancy
Respiratory problems (See Acute breathlessness)				
Perimenopause/Menopause (See Night sweats)				
Post-traumatic stress disorder	History of a recent threatening or catastrophic event Involves oneself or others Recurrent and chronic symptoms High-risk groups: Elderly, children, veterans, mental health patients, refugees	Recurrent flashbacks of the event Difficulty falling or staying asleep Nightmares Avoidance of situations likely to trigger memories Loss of interest in other activities Jumpy and easily startled Increased vigilance Low mood Poor concentration Loss of libido	Persistent fear and anxiety Depression ± Drug or alcohol abuse	Risk of: Alcohol and drug abuse, somatisation, chronic pain and poor health

Night sweats

Diagnosis	Background	Key symptoms	Key signs	Additional information
Perimenopause/Menopause	Menopause occurs ≈50 yrs age Premature if onset <40 yrs age Preceded by the climacteric Elevated FSH and LH Low oestradiol Symptoms can persist for years	*Climacteric:* Irregular menses (short or long cycles) Menorrhagia Hot flushes Night sweats Palpitations Vaginal dryness Urinary frequency Stress incontinence Low mood or anxiety Insomnia Reduced libido *Menopause:* *As above plus:* Secondary amenorrhoea for ≥12 months	Dry skin Thinning hair Atrophic vaginitis	Risk of: Osteoporosis, IHD, cerebrovascular disease Postmenopausal bleeding is abnormal if present, refer to exclude endometrial carcinoma

Diagnosis	Background	Key symptoms	Key signs	Additional information
Pulmonary tuberculosis **Stage of infection:**	Chronic granulomatous disease Droplet spread			Notifiable disease Refer to respiratory specialist

Primary TB	Initial infection produces a
	   pulmonary lesion (Ghon focus)
	Ghon focus usually heals and
	   calcifies
	Immunity develops
		Usually asymptomatic or
		Non-specific (e.g. fatigue, weight
		   loss)
			Signs may be absent	Complications include
				   widespread dissemination of TB
				   (Miliary TB)

Post-primary TB	Reactivation of primary TB
	Ghon focus enlarges with
	   lymphatic spread
	± Extra-pulmonary organ spread
	   (e.g. bone)
	Risk factors: Close contact
	   with TB patient, children,
	   vagrants, foreign travel,
	   immunocompromise,
	   malnutrition
		Symptoms develop late:
		Productive cough
		Fatigue
		Weight loss
		Anorexia
		Night sweats
		± Haemoptysis
			Fever
			Cervical LN
			Variable respiratory signs
			± Erythema nodosum
				Respiratory signs vary (e.g. upper
				   lobe crackles, effusion)
				Complications include
				   widespread dissemination of TB
				   (Miliary TB)

Infective endocarditis	Affects normal or abnormal
	   valves
	Infection is acute in normal valves
	   and subacute in abnormal
	   valves
	M:F ratio: ≈3:1
	Risk factors: Invasive vascular
	   procedures, i.v. drug use,
	   gingivitis, rheumatic fever,
	   abnormal or prosthetic valves
	Mitral valve and aortic valve are
	   usually affected
	Commonest pathogen:
	   Staphylococcus aureus
	Vegetations can cause valve
	   destruction, regurgitation or
	   obstruction
	Associated with vasculitis and
	   arterial emboli
		Rigors
		Night sweats
		Malaise
		Weight loss
			Fever
			Anaemia
			Generalised petechial rash
			New valvular regurgitation or
			A changing pre-existing murmur
			Clubbing
			Splenomegaly
			Arthritis
			Meningitis
			Roth spots (retinal haemorrhages)
			Splinter (subungual)
			   haemorrhages:
			Linear red lines parallel with
			   longaxis of the nail
			Affects finger or toe nails
			Osler's nodes:
			Tender red/purple pulp nodules
			Affects finger or toes
			Janeway lesions:
			Painless erythematous macules
			Affects palms
				Emergency admission
				Common complications: CCF,
				   aortic valve insufficiency,
				   arterial emboli

Lymphoma **Subtypes:**				

Non-Hodgkin's	Five times more common than
	   Hodgkin's lymphoma
	Commonly presents >50 yrs age
	M<F
	Disease may originate from
	   extranodal sites (e.g. GI, skin,
	   chest)
		Often asymptomatic or
		Presents like Hodgkin's
			Anaemia
			Painless LN enlargement
			Hepatosplenomegaly	

Hodgkin's	Young adults and elderly
	M:F ratio: ≈2:1
	Risk factors: History of
	   infectious mononucleosis, HIV,
	   immunosupression, smoking
		A symptoms:
		Asymptomatic or pruritis
		B symptoms:
		Chronic weight loss >10% in 6
		   months
		Fever
		Night sweats
			Cachexia
			Anaemia
			Painless LN enlargement (neck,
			   axillae, supraclavicular)
			Hepatosplenomegaly
				B symptoms indicates more
				   extensive disease

Diagnosis	Background	Key symptoms	Key signs	Additional information
Chronic myeloid leukaemia	Abnormal proliferation of haemopoietic stem cell line(s) Commonly age >60 yrs Associated with Philadelphia chromosome Quiescent for years before rapid onset myeloproliferation	Insidious onset Spontaneous bruising Fatigue Weight loss Night sweats Abdominal fullness LUQ pain (splenic infarction)	Fever Anaemia Petechiae Local or generalised LN Abdominal distension Hepatosplenomegaly Gout (rapid cell turnover) Hyperviscosity syndrome (e.g. CVA) ± Bruises	
Malaria	Usually *Plasmodium falciparum* The most severe Plasmodium strain Causes haemolytic anaemia Incubation 7–14 days Usually presents within 2 months Endemic areas: SE Asia, Far East, sub-Saharan Africa Risk factors: Recent travel, airport staff	Recurrent fever Malaise Headache Anorexia Myalgia *Followed by:* Rigors Night sweats	Fever Anaemia Hepatosplenomegaly	Notifiable disease Warrants emergency admission Complications include: Cerebral malaria, hypoglycaemia, severe anaemia, pulmonary oedema, acute renal failure A single negative blood film does not exclude malaria
Human immunodeficiency virus (HIV) (See Weight loss)				

Syncope (Blackouts)

Diagnosis	Background	Key symptoms	Key signs	Additional information
Vasovagal attack	Neurally mediated syncope Causes abnormal vasodilatation, hypotension and bradycardia Trigger factors: Emotion, heat, pain, fear, prolonged standing No underlying cardiac disease Quickly relieved or prevented by lying down	*Prodromal symptoms:* Sweating Nausea Lower limb weakness Closing of vision Dizziness No chest pain	Syncope lasts up to 2 mins Rapid recovery post-syncope No amnesia or confusion No tonic–clonic limb movements Normal blood pressure No focal neurology No post-ictal phase	
Hypoglycaemia	Possible history of pre-existing or undiagnosed DM Causes: Insulin/oral hypoglycaemics, sulfonylurea, alcohol binge, pituitary insufficiency, liver failure, Addison's disease, insulinoma, post gastric surgery	Lethargy Sweating Hunger Tremor Paraesthesia in lips and tongue Poor concentration	Apyrexial No cyanosis Finger-prick BM <3.0 mmol/litre Slurred speech ± Transient hemiplegia (rarely in IDDM) ± LoC	
Heart block (Atrioventricular block)	Conduction defect of the AV node and/or Bundle of His No trigger factors		Confirmation of diagnosis on ECG Cardiovascular examination may be normal	
Subtypes:				
First degree	Slow AV node conduction Atrial impulses are conducted to ventricles PR interval >0.2 secs Benign Associated with: CAD, rheumatic fever, digitalis toxicity, electrolyte imbalance	Asymptomatic	Regular pulse	

Diagnosis	Background	Key symptoms	Key signs	Additional information
Types of second-degree heart block:	Some atrial impulses fail to conduct to the ventricles			
Mobitz Type I (Wenckebach phenomenon)	AV node conduction defect Progressive lengthening of PR interval followed by a dropped atrial beat Usually benign	Missed beats	Regularly irregular pulse	
Mobitz Type II	Conduction defect below AV node Constant PR interval with occasional atrial dropped beat Risk of third-degree heart block	Dizziness Syncope	Irregularly irregular pulse	Refer to cardiology
2:1 block	Alternate conducted and non-conducted atrial beats Constant PR interval in conducted beats Risk factors: Digitalis toxicity, myocardial ischaemia Risk of third-degree heart block	Dizziness Syncope	Regular pulse	Refer to cardiology
Third-degree heart block (Complete heart block)	AV dissociation Ventricles contract via an escape rhythm No relationship between P and QRS waves Commonly elderly Causes: Myocardial fibrosis, inferior MI, digitalis posioning, sick sinus syndrome, bundle branch block	Intermittent syncope (Stoke-Adams attacks) White appearance presyncope Disorientation Fatigue Shortness of breath	Facial flushing on recovery Regular heart rate <50 bpm Hypotension Tachypnoea Raised JVP Intermittent cannon A waves ± Heart failure	Urgent admission for a pacemaker
Epilepsy	Partial or generalised seizures Partial seizures affect one part of hemisphere Generalised seizures affect both hemispheres Causes: Idiopathic, SOL, infection, metabolic abnormality (e.g. hypernatraemia), CVA, head trauma, drugs Triggers: Sleep deprivation, alcohol, medication (e.g. TCA)	± History of prodromal symptoms (e.g. change in mood/behaviour)		Status epilepticus requires emergency admission Consider further investigation in any unprovoked seizure Hepatic enzyme-inducing anti-epileptics interact with the COCP and POP Advise against driving and patient to inform DVLA
Common subtypes:				
Temporal lobe epilepsy	Partial seizure Can be simple or complex Simple partial seizure: No LoC ± aura Complex partial: LoC	*Preceding aura: lasts ≈2 mins* Visual (e.g. distortion of shapes) Olfactory Gustatory Auditory (e.g. vertigo) Psychic (e.g. déjà vu) Autonomic (e.g. sweating)	*During seizure:* Motionless wide-eyed stare Dilated pupils Lip smacking Unilateral dystonic limb posture ± LoC *Post-ictal:* Confusion Amnesia (if complex seizure)	Complex partial seizures can become generalised Todds paralysis: After a partial seizure, there may be temporary weakness of the affected limb
Absences (Petit mal)	Generalised seizure Onset in childhood Seizure starts and ends abruptly Up to 100 episodes/day may occur Often remits in adulthood	Acute episodes of staring spells No aura	Absences last ≤10 secs ± Clonic movements of arms No post-ictal confusion	

Diagnosis	Background	Key symptoms	Key signs	Additional information
Tonic–clonic epilepsy (Grand mal)	Generalised seizure	Preceding aura Sudden collapse with LoC Jerking of limbs witnessed	*During seizure:* Bilateral limbs stiffen (tonic) Bilateral limbs jerk (clonic) ± Bladder incontinence ± Tongue biting *Post ictal:* Acute confusion Headache Reduced level of consciousness Poor short term memory	
Myoclonic epilepsy	Generalised seizure Peak onset age 6–10 yrs Associated with epileptogenic photosensitvity	Typical onset 1 h after waking Sudden jerks Often involves arms or trunk	Examination often unremarkable	
Infantile spasms	Generalised seizure Commonly age 3–8 months Causes: Idiopathic, birth hypoxia, congenital infection, hypoglycaemia, tuberous sclerosis, meningitis, encephalitis, Often results in cogntive impairment and cerebral palsy	Frequent seizures every 10–15 secs Seizures last a few seconds	*During seizure:* Rigid trunk Symmetrical flexing of arms ± Limb extension or absences	
Febrile convulsions	Generalised seizure Benign Occurs in a developmentally normal child Commonly age 6 months to 5 yrs Triggered by fever Associated with extra-cranial infection (e.g. URTI) High recurrence	Unwell child Seizure lasts <10 mins	Fever *During seizure:* Generalised trunk stiffness Shaking all over Eyes roll up ± Bladder incontinence *Post-ictal:* Reduced level of consciousness No persistent neurological deficit	Consider meningitis and encephalitis
Cerebral vascular accident or TIA (See Dysphagia)				
Myocardial infarction	M>F Risk factors: Advancing age, family history, South Asian, obesity, hyperlipidaemia, DM, smoking, hypertension	Acute onset Central heavy crushing chest pain Or epigastric pain ± Radiation to neck, jaw, arm(s) Duration >20 mins Not relieved by rest or GTN Nausea Sweating Shortness of breath Collapse	Low-grade fever <39°C Anxiety Cold and clammy Systolic murmur ± Heart failure ± Loss of consciousness	Beware of silent MI in the elderly or diabetic. Symptoms are often atypical
Situational syncope	Neurally mediated syncope Causes abnormal vasodilatation, hypotension and bradycardia Common triggers: Micturition, coughing, defaecation, heavy meals No underlying cardiac disease	Long-standing history of syncope Occurs during or immediately after certain triggers Prodromal dizziness Followed by syncope Headache and nausea post-syncope No chest pain No amnesia or confusion	No focal neurology	

Diagnosis	Background	Key symptoms	Key signs	Additional information
White breath-holding attacks	Reflex asystolic or bradycardic attacks Benign Presents in infants or children aged <4 yrs Precipitated by pain or shock (e.g. injury, fall) Attacks often spontaneously resolve by age 4 yrs	Brief episode of crying Followed by breath holding Pallor Collapse Transient bradycardia or cardiac arrest ± LoC ± Tonic–clonic seizures	Examination unremarkable	
Aortic stenosis (See Dizziness)				
Carotid sinus hypersensitivity	Transient asystole >3 secs and/or hypotension Triggered by pressure on carotid sinus (e.g. tumour, shaving, tight collar) Commonly age >50 yrs M>F Risk factors: CAD, hypertension, Lewy body dementia, drugs (e.g. beta-blockers)	Acute onset syncope Typically follows head turning	Normal blood pressure on recovery No tonic–clonic limb movements witnessed No post-ictal confusion	Consider cardiology referral
Narcolepsy	Chronic neurological sleep disorder Overwhelming desire to sleep Typical onset in adolescence M>F Strong genetic component Associated with: Major stress, pregnancy, head trauma	Daily symptoms Irresistible attacks of inappropriate daytime sleep Triggered by emotion ± Vivid hallucinations, worse on falling asleep or waking ± Transient generalised sleep paralysis on waking ± Cataplexy (acute loss of muscle power and tone)	Examination unremarkable	Exclude insomnia and sedatives

Tremor

Diagnosis	Background	Key symptoms	Key signs	Additional information
Generalised anxiety disorder	Usually chronic and persistent anxiety Excessive or unrealistic worry Inappropriate to the situation Affects daily functioning Associated with stress and depression	Fast palpitations Shortness of breath Dizziness Nausea/vomiting Numbness and tingling "Fear of losing control" Poor concentration Insomnia Urinary frequency Frequent or loose bowel motions Erectile dysfunction	Hyperventilation Sweating Sinus tachycardia Hypertension Severe anxiety Fear of death/illness Postural hand tremor	Exclude alcohol/drug misuse
Delerium tremens (See Acute confusion)				
Benign essential tremor	Progressive postural tremor Strong familial tendency Variable in severity	Initially unilateral upper limb tremor Progresses to involve both arms ± Neck and facial muscles Can be worse with emotion Often relieved by alcohol No tremor during sleep	Systemically well Persistent postural tremor Mildly asymmetrical Able to exert some control during concentrated activity Normal neurological examination	Risk of depression and alcoholism

Diagnosis	Background	Key symptoms	Key signs	Additional information
Parkinson's disease	Idiopathic movement disorder Degeneration of substantia nigra dopaminergic neurones Degenerating neurones contain Lewy bodies Peak onset 55–65 yrs age Other causes of parkinsonism: Drug-induced (e.g. neuroleptics), post-encephalitis, toxins, head trauma, Wilson's disease, Lewy body dementia, vascular dementia	Recurrent falls with no LoC Resting tremor Worse with stress Relieved by voluntary movement Dysphagia and dribbling Low mood in ≈50%	Festinated (shuffling steps) gait Unilateral resting "pill rolling" tremor Generalised tremor years later Bradykinesia Expressionless face Monotonous speech Cogwheel or lead-pipe rigidity during passive limb movement Present in flexors and extensors Micrographia Normal muscle power Normal tendon reflexes Normal plantar responses	Late onset dementia may develop after ≈10 yrs
Drug-induced tremor	Common drugs: TCA, salbutamol, antipsychotics, lithium, sodium valproate, metaclopramide, theophylline, alcohol, illict drugs	Onset postural tremor after taking medication	Normal neurological examination	Exclude excess caffeine and recent drug withdrawal
Hyperthyroidism (Thyrotoxicosis)	Primary or secondary Age 20–50 yrs M:F ratio: ≈1:9 Causes: Graves' disease, thyroiditis, toxic nodule, amiodarone Eye changes suggest Graves' disease (e.g. exophthalmos)	Fast palpitations Hyperactivity Sweating Weight loss despite increased appetite Diarrhoea Heat intolerance ± Oligo/amenorrhoea	Tachycardia Lid lag Hair thinning or alopecia Fine postural hand tremor Warm peripheries Gynaecomastia Neck lump Lump moves up on swallowing Brisk reflexes ± AF ± Dull percussion over sternum ± Psychosis	Consider thyrotoxic crisis if: Fever Delirium Coma Seizures Jaundice Vomiting
Type II respiratory failure	Low oxygen and carbon dioxide retention Causes: COPD, pneumonia, pulmonary fibrosis, sedative drugs, CNS tumour, CNS trauma, sepsis, diaphragmatic paralysis, myasthenia gravis, Guillain-Barré, kyphoscoliosis	*Hypoxia:* Shortness of breath Exhaustion Agitation *Hypercapnia:* Headache Drowsiness	*Hypoxia:* Central cyanosis Confusion Tachypnoea *Hypercapnia:* Confusion Tachyardia Peripheral vasodilatation Bounding radial pulse Flapping hand tremor Papilloedema	Oxygen therapy should be given with care as respiration may be driven by hypoxia
Liver failure (See Chronic confusion)				
Cerebellar ataxia	Failure of voluntary muscle co-ordination despite normal power Commonest causes: Wernicke's encephalopathy and Friedreich's ataxia Other causes: Developmental, infectious, MS, neoplastic, vascular	Unable to walk in a straight line Worse in the dark Clumsiness in carrying objects	*Signs of cerebellar dysfunction:* Dysarthria Ataxic gait Unable to tandem walk (heel to toe) Nystagmus (eye drift towards side of lesion with rapid correction) Hypotonia Incoordination in finger–nose test Incoordination in heel–kneel–shin test Intention tremor on movement Dysdiadochokinesis	Signs are ipsilateral to the side of hemispheric damage

Weight gain

Diagnosis	Background	Key symptoms	Key signs	Additional information
Idiopathic weight gain	Common risk factors: Family history, inactivity, diet, social deprivation, alcohol abuse Associated with: IHD, hypertension, Type II DM, sleep apnoea, endometrial carcinoma, infertility, osteoarthritis, increase oestrogen	Weight gain can be rapid or gradual Breathlessness on exertion	BMI >25 kg/m² Pseudogynaecomastia Normal respiratory examination	
Metabolic syndrome (Syndrome X)	Defined by ≥3 of the following: Truncal obesity Elevated triglycerides Decreased HDL cholesterol Hypertension Impaired glucose tolerance Risk factors: Insulin resistance, obesity, inactivity, fatty diet Associated with: CHD, Type II DM, chronic kidney disease, fatty liver, PCOS	Often asymptomatic	Hypertension Truncal obesity	
Premenstrual tension syndrome	Symptom-free for at least 1 wk per cycle Pre-existing psychiatric conditions often made worse Risk factors: Obesity, smoking, poor diet, lack of exercise	Cyclical symptoms Lasts days/weeks before menses Relieved shortly after onset of menses Headache Irritable Anxiety Low mood Abdominal bloating Breast tenderness Aching legs	Normal abdominal examination No depression or hypomania	
Peripheral oedema	Causes inlcude: Pregnancy, cardiac failure, renal failure, ascites	Symptoms vary depending on underlying cause Swelling is gradual	Signs vary depending on underlying cause Pitting oedema	Ascites may indicate underlying malignancy
Polycystic ovarian syndrome	Pre-menopausal women Associated with insulin resistance and infertility ≥2 of the following: Symptomatic Elevated LH (or FSH during menses) and supressed SHBG Polycystic ovaries on ultrasound	Asymptomatic or Irregular or absent menses Excess body hair Frontal balding	± BMI >30 kg/m² ± Acne ± Hirsutism	Weight loss is beneficial
Acquired hypothyroidism	Age >60 yrs M<F Causes: Autoimmune, thyroiditis, TSH deficiency, postpartum, thyroidectomy, neck radiation, iodine deficiency, drugs (e.g. amiodarone, carbizamole) Associated with high cholesterol/triglycerides and anaemia	Lethargy Constipation Low mood Cold intolerance Menorrhagia	Deep hoarse voice Slow cognition (e.g. poor memory) Dry coarse skin Thinning of hair Bradycardia Slow-relaxing tendon reflexes ± Goitre	Beware myxoedema in the elderly: Puffy eyes, hands and feet Cerebellar ataxia Hypothermia Seizures ± Coma
Medication	Common drugs: Gliclazide, steroids, insulin, oestrogen, atypical antipsychotics, antiretroviral	Onset of weight gain after taking medication	Weight gain	

Diagnosis	Background	Key symptoms	Key signs	Additional information
Cushing's syndrome	Causes: Cushing's disease, iatrogenic glucocorticoid excess, adrenal tumour, small cell lung carcinoma Commonly 30–50 yrs age M<F Associated with osteoporosis	Increase in abdominal girth Irregular menses or amenorrhoea Excess body hair Easy bruising Impotence	Hypertension Moon face Acne Interscapular fat pad (buffalo hump) Purple/red abdominal striae Truncal obesity Thin pigmented skin Hirsutism Proximal muscle weakness	
Nephrotic syndrome	Glomerular dysfunction causes excessive urinary protein excretion Results in proteinuria, hypoalbuminaemia and oedema Common causes: Glomerulonephritis (commonly minimal change GN), post-infection (e.g. Group A beta haemolytic streptococci, hepatitis B), collagen vascular disease (e.g. SLE), DM, myeloma, drugs (e.g. NSAID)	Fatigue Poor appetite Frothy urine	Facial swelling (in children) Periorbital oedema (in children) Peripheral lower-limb oedema May become generalised Xanthelasma Xanthomata ± Hypertension ± Pleural effusion *Abnormal urinalysis:* Gross proteinuria ± Haematuria	Consider urgent nephrology referral Complications: Reduced resistance to infection, thromboembolism, hyperlipidaemia, ARF

Weight loss

Diagnosis	Background	Key symptoms	Key signs	Additional information
Acute stress	Acute physical or emotional stress Emotional stresses include: Exams, new job, divorce, redundancy, bereavement, moving house Usually resolves with time	History of recent stressful event Reduced appetite Mild anxiety Low mood Insomnia ± Secondary amenorrhoea	Systemically well No depression	Secondary amenorrhoea common in athletes Amenorrhoea increases risk of osteoporosis
Diabetes mellitus	Predisposing factors for DKA or HONK: Any infection, inadequate insulin or non-compliance, undiagnosed DM, illness (e.g. MI, CVA), drugs (e.g. beta-blockers, diuretics)			Patient should inform DVLA Complications: CVA, MI, retinopathy, limb ischaemia, neuropathy, infections
Subtypes:				
Type I diabetes	Lack of endogenous insulin Commonly children or young adults Genetic predisposition Associated with autoimmune disease Risk of ketoacidosis Presentation is acute or subacute Longer history of symptoms	*Acute diabetic ketoacidosis:* Acute onset symptoms Fatigue Malaise Weight loss Polyuria and frequency Polydipsia Nausea/vomiting Non-specific abdominal pain *Subacute symptoms:* Fatigue Weight loss Polyuria and frequency Polydipsia Plus recurrent infections (e.g. boils, thrush, UTI)	*Acute diabetic ketoacidosis:* Severe dehydration Tachycardia Tachypnoea Ketotic breath ± Confusion ± Infection (e.g. URTI, UTI) *Abnormal urinalysis:* Glucose Ketones *Subacute signs:* *Abnormal urinalysis:* Glucose ± Ketones	DKA warrants emergency admission

Diagnosis	Background	Key symptoms	Key signs	Additional information
Type II diabetes	Reduced insulin secretion Increased insulin resistance Typical age >40 yrs Commonest type of diabetes Common risk factors: Obesity, South Asian, Afro-Caribbean, male gender, family history, gestational DM, impaired glucose tolerance, metabolic syndrome, drugs (e.g. steroids) Not prone to ketoacidosis Presents insidiously or subacutely with HONK	*Insidious onset:* Weight loss Polyuria and frequency Polydipsia *Hyperosmolar non-ketotic coma:* Gradual onset symptoms over ≥1 wk Generalised weakness Lethargy ± Seizures	*Insidious onset:* Few signs may be present Glycosuria *Hyperosmolar non-ketotic coma:* Severe dehydration Tachycardia Confusion Drowsy Finger-prick glucose >30 mmol/litre ± Focal CNS signs (e.g. hemiparesis) ± Infection *Abnormal urinalyis:* Glucose No ketones	May eventually require insulin HONK warrants emergency admission High risk of DVT
Hyperthyroidism (Thyrotoxicosis)	Primary or secondary Age 20–50 yrs M:F ratio: ≈1:9 Causes: Graves' disease, thyroiditis, toxic nodule, amiodarone Eye changes suggest Graves' disease (e.g. exophthalmos)	Fast palpitations Hyperactivity Sweating Weight loss despite increase appetite Diarrhoea Heat intolerance ± Oligo/amenorrhoea	Tachycardia Lid lag Hair thinning or alopecia Fine postural hand tremor Warm peripheries Gynaecomastia Neck lump Neck lump moves up on swallowing Brisk reflexes ± AF ± Dull percussion over sternum ± Psychosis	Consider thyrotoxic crisis if: Fever Delirium Coma Seizures Jaundice Vomiting
Malignancy	A common cause of bone pain Often suggests metastatic disease	Back, rib or hip pain Worse at night Weight loss Malaise *Symptoms of hypercalcaemia:* Lethargy Low mood Polyuria Polydipsia Constipation Muscle weakness	Bony tenderness Occasional soft tissue masses Gradual progressive neuropathy Hepatomegaly Pathological fractures	
Rheumatoid arthritis (See Hand and wrist pain)				
Crohns' disease (See Diarrhoea)				
Chronic pancreatitis	Irreversible pancreatic fibrosis Results in malabsorption and DM Causes include: Alcohol (≈60%), pancreatic duct obstruction, cystic fibrosis, haemochromotosis, hypercalcaemia, drugs, trauma	Chronic or intermittent epigastric pain Often severe Radiates through to back Relieved by sitting forward Steatorrhoea Anorexia Weight loss Nausea/vomiting	Mild or moderate epigastric tenderness	Pain is a common complication Beware opiate addiction
Pulmonary tuberculosis (See Cough)				

Diagnosis	Background	Key symptoms	Key signs	Additional information
Depression	Risk factors: Genetic, lower social class Precipitating factors include: Bereavement, job loss, relationship break-up, chronic illness, drugs (e.g. beta-blockers) May be part of Bipolar disorder	Low mood or anhedonia Lasts most of the day for most days Loss of appetite Weight loss Insomnia Early morning awakening Persistent fatigue Loss of libido Feeling worthless or guilty Poor concentration	Expressionless face Tearful Apathy Uncommunicative Self-neglect Psychomotor retardation Deliberate self-harm Suicidal ideation or intent	Consider hospital admission in severe cases or risk of suicide
Anorexia nervosa	BMI <17.5 kg/m² Deliberate weight loss Restricted food intake Typical onset mid-adolescence M:F ratio: ≈1:10 Distorted body image Risk factors: Cultural, occupational demands (e.g. modelling, dancing) Associated with: Over-exercise, laxative and diuretic abuse, bulimia	Rapid and severe weight loss "Fear of putting on weight" Low mood Social withdrawal	Bradycardia Hypotension Hypothermia Cachexia Distorted body image Preoccupation with food Depression ± Dental enamel erosion ± Lanugo hair growth	Complications include: Cardiac failure, renal failure, osteoporosis Risk of suicide
Bulimia nervosa	BMI may be normal Typical onset adolescence or young adulthood M:F ratio: ≈1:10 Distorted body image Risk factors: Previous obesity, dieting, sexual/physical abuse, stressful life events (e.g. parental death) Associated with: Over-exercise, laxative and diuretic abuse, substance abuse, fasting	Recurrent symptoms "Fear of putting on weight" Uncontrolled overeating (binges) Followed by guilt and self-induced vomiting Triggered by boredom, loneliness, rejection Low mood Social withdrawal	Dental enamel erosion Distorted body image Preoccupation with food Depression	Complications include: Metabolic alkalosis, renal failure, cardiac arrhythmias Risk of suicide
Human immunodeficiency virus (HIV)	Retrovirus binds to CD4 receptors Integrates DNA copy of RNA genome into host DNA and replicates HIV risk factors: Unprotected vaginal or anal sex, contaminated needle use, contaminated blood contact, perinatal transmission (including breastfeeding)			Consider a full sexual health screen HIV testing requires informed consent and counselling HIV tests should be performed 3–6 months post-exposure. A positive result should be repeated
Stages of infection:				
Acute infection and seroconversion	Seroconversion occurs 2–6 wks post-infection Results in viraemia and HIV dissemination Symptoms often resolve within 2 wks	Initially asymptomatic *Followed by seroconversion:* Malaise Myalgia Sore throat	*Seroconversion:* Fever Generalised LN Pharyngitis Generalised maculopapular rash ± Aseptic meningitis (rare)	
Asymptomatic	Rapid viral replication	Asymptomatic	Normal examination or Generalised LN >1 cm diameter Symmetrical LN LN for >3 months	

Diagnosis	Background	Key symptoms	Key signs	Additional information
Non-specific constitutional symptoms	Infections tend to be recurrent and severe	Minor recurrent occult infections (e.g. oral candidiasis, seborrhoeic dermatitis, shingles) Night sweats Diarrhoea Weight loss	Fever Focal infection	
Acquired immunodeficiency syndrome (AIDS)	Characterised by ≥1 opportunistic infections or malignancies CD4 count <200 × 10^6/L Common opportunistic infections: PCP, cerebral toxoplasmosis, oesophageal candidiasis, cryptosporidium or CMV diarrhoea Common malignancies: Kaposi's sarcoma, invasive cervical carcinoma, B-cell non-Hodgkin's lymphoma	Vary depending on underlying infection or malignancy	Vary depending on underlying infection or malignancy	

Index